SOS
Safe Obstetric Systems

Making Obstetrics Safer
FETAL PILLOW
www.fetalpillow.com

Designed to make second stage Caesarean Sections easier, safer and less traumatic

Fetal Pillow use in a prospective randomised study of 240_{pts} shows significant improvements in maternal outcomes when used in a Caesarean Section at full dilation.

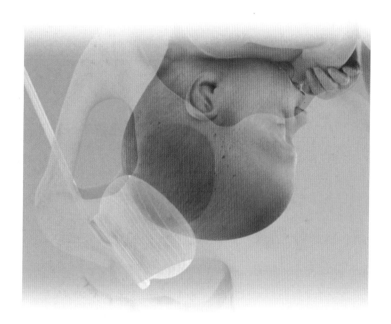

- Reduced Uterine Extensions
- Reduction in Total Operating Time
- Reduction in Incision to Delivery Time
- Reduced Blood Loss
- Reduction in need for Blood Transfusion

SAFE OBSTETRIC SYSTEMS LTD

1. EP1.414 Reducing complications in a caesarean section at full dilation using fetal pillow: a prospective randomised trial. Seal, S; Barman, SC; Tibriwal, R; De, A; Kanrar, P; Mukherjii, J. BJOG. Volume 120. Issue Supplement s1. 21 June 2013.

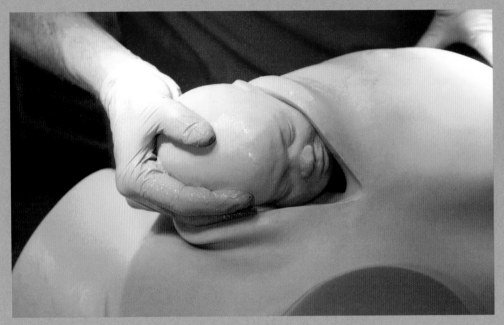
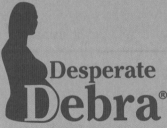
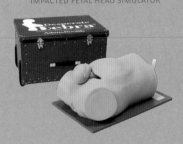

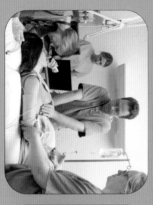
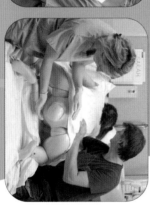
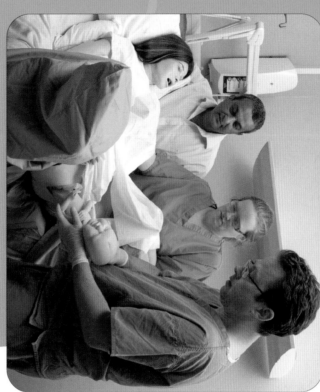
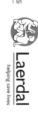

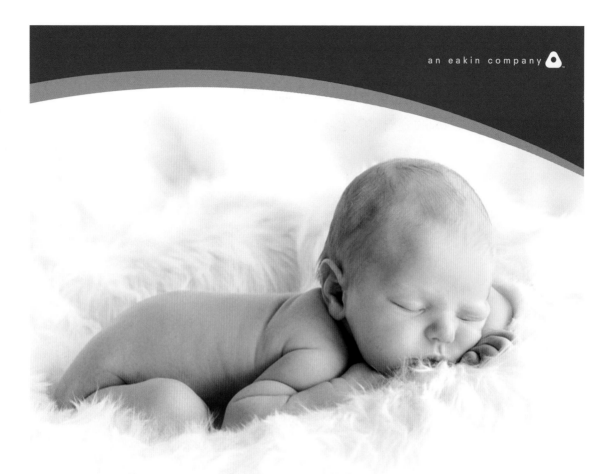
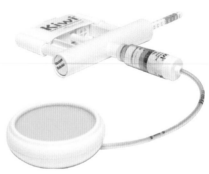
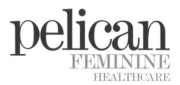

ROBuST
RCOG Operative Birth Simulation Training

ROBuST

RCOG Operative Birth Simulation Training

Course Manual

Edited by

George Attilakos, Tim Draycott, Alison Gale,
Dimitrios Siassakos and Cathy Winter

CAMBRIDGE
UNIVERSITY PRESS

University Printing House, Cambridge CB2 8BS, United Kingdom

Published in the United States of America by Cambridge University Press, New York

Cambridge University Press is part of the University of Cambridge.

It furthers the University's mission by disseminating knowledge in the pursuit of
education, learning and research at the highest international levels of excellence.

www.cambridge.org
Information on this title: www.cambridge.org/9781107680302

© Cambridge University Press 2014

First published 2014

Printed in the United Kingdom by Bell and Bain Ltd

A catalogue record for this publication is available from the British Library

Library of Congress Cataloging-in-Publication Data
ROBuST : RCOG operative birth simulation training / edited by George Attilakos, Tim Draycott, Alison Gale, Dimitrios Siassakos,
Cathy Winter.
      p. ; cm.
RCOG operative birth simulation training
Operative birth simulation training
Includes bibliographical references and index.
ISBN 978-1-107-68030-2 (Paperback : alk. paper)
I. Attilakos, George, editor of compilation.   II. Gale, Alison (Obstetrician), editor of compilation.   III. Siassakos, Dimitrios,
editor of compilation.   IV. Draycott, Timothy J., editor of compilation.   V. Winter, Cathy (Midwife), editor of
compilation.   VI. Royal College of Obstetricians and Gynaecologists (Great Britain), issuing body.   VII. Title: RCOG operative
birth simulation training.   VIII. Title: Operative birth simulation training.
[DNLM: 1. Extraction, Obstetrical–methods.   2. Extraction, Obstetrical–adverse effects. WQ 415]
RG725
618.8–dc23   2013035743

ISBN 978-1-107-68030-2 Paperback

Every effort has been made in preparing this book to provide accurate and up-to-date information which is in accord with
accepted standards and practice at the time of publication. Although case histories are drawn from actual cases, every effort has
been made to disguise the identities of the individuals involved. Nevertheless, the authors, editors and publishers can make no
warranties that the information contained herein is totally free from error, not least because clinical standards are constantly
changing through research and regulation. The authors, editors and publishers therefore disclaim all liability for direct or
consequential damages resulting from the use of material contained in this book. Readers are strongly advised to pay careful
attention to information provided by the manufacturer of any drugs or equipment that they plan to use.

Contents

Contributors

Mr George Attilakos	Consultant Obstetrician, London
Dr Rachna Bahl	Consultant Obstetrician, Bristol
Dr Sadia Bhatti	Consultant Obstetrician, Twickenham
Dr Jennifer Browne	Specialty Trainee in Obstetrics and Gynaecology
Dr George Bugg	Consultant Obstetrician, Nottingham
Dr Katie Cornthwaite	Specialty Trainee in Obstetrics and Gynaecology
Dr Fiona Day	Specialty Trainee in Obstetrics and Gynaecology
Prof Timothy Draycott	Consultant Obstetrician, Bristol
Dr Alison Gale	Consultant Obstetrician and Gynaecologist, Preston Simulation Advisor to RCOG
Mr Kim Hinshaw	Consultant Obstetrician and Gynaecologist, Sunderland
Dr Tamara Kubba	Specialty Trainee in Obstetrics and Gynaecology
Dr David Levy	Consultant Anaesthetist, Nottingham
Dr Shilpa Mahadasu	Specialty Trainee in Obstetrics and Gynaecology
Dr Fraser McLeod	Consultant Obstetrician and Gynaecologist, Bristol
Dr Rasha Mohammed	Specialty Trainee in Obstetrics and Gynaecology
Professor Glen Mola	Professor of Obstetrics and Gynecology, School of Medicine and Health Sciences, University of Papua New Guinea
Professor Deirdre Murphy	Head of Obstetrics and Gynaecology, Trinity College, University of Dublin
Dr Sarah Newell	Specialty Trainee in Obstetrics and Gynaecology

Mr Patrick O'Brien	Consultant Obstetrician and Gynaecologist, London
Mr Karl Oláh	Consultant Obstetrician and Gynaecologist, Warwick
Dr Matthew Prior	Specialty Trainee in Obstetrics and Gynaecology RCOG Trainees' Committee Representative
Dr Rowena Pykett	Specialty Trainee in Obstetrics and Gynaecology
Dr Meenakshi Ramphul	Consultant Obstetrician and Gynaecologist, Dublin
Dr Dimitrios Siassakos	Clinical Lecturer, University of Bristol
Dr Priya Sokhal	Specialty Trainee in Obstetrics and Gynaecology
Dr Bryony Strachan	Consultant Obstetrician and Gynaecologist, Bristol
Dr Aldo Vacca	Consultant Obstetrician, Brisbane
Dr Helen van der Nelson	Specialty Trainee in Obstetrics and Gynaecology
Ms Cathy Winter	PRactical Obstetric Multi-Professional Training (PROMPT) Maternity Foundation Research Midwife

Acknowledgements

The editors would like to thank the Product Development and Marketing Executive of the Royal College of Obstetricians and Gynaecologists (RCOG) who accepted the proposal for this educational text and course.

We are grateful to the individual chapter authors for sharing their expert knowledge and skills in the production of the core text and training course.

We acknowledge the work of Claire Dunn, RCOG Publishing, without whom this project would not have been possible.

We would also like to show our gratitude to the trainees who contributed to the development of the course:

- Matthew Prior – RCOG trainee representative
- Rasha Mohammed
- Jennifer Browne
- Sarah Newell
- Helen van der Nelson
- Fiona Day
- Katie Cornthwaite
- Tamara Kubba
- Priya Sokhal

Finally, we would like to thank all the trainers who will deliver this training course on behalf of RCOG in the future.

George Attilakos, Tim Draycott, Alison Gale, Dimitrios Siassakos and Cathy Winter

Abbreviations

ACOG .... American College of Obstetricians and Gynecologists
BMI .... body mass index
BPD .... biparietal diameter
CEFM .... continuous electronic fetal monitoring
CPD.................... cephalopelvic disproportion
CS .... caesarean section
CSF.................... cerebrospinal fluid
CTG.................... cardiotocography
DDI..................... decision to delivery interval
DOA .... direct occipito-anterior
DOP.................... direct occipito-posterior
EFM.................... electronic fetal monitoring
FBS .... fetal blood samples
GA .... general anaesthesia
HIE .... hypoxic-ischaemic encephalopathy
ICU..................... intensive care unit
ITU .... infrapubic translabial ultrasound
LA .... local anaesthetic
NHSLA................ National Health Service Litigation Authority
NICE .... National Institute for Health and Care Excellence
OA .... occipito-anterior
OP...................... occipito-posterior
OT .... occipito-transverse
OVB.................... operative vaginal birth
RCOG................. Royal College of Obstetricians and Gynaecologists
VTE..................... venous thromboembolism
WHO .... World Health Organization

Preface

In order to ensure we provide the highest quality of care to women, RCOG sets high standards in training. The emphasis is to ensure that the future specialists acquire both technical and non-technical skills, which together are essential to correctly manage patients within a well-functioning team of professionals. Providing training with these aims is at the forefront of RCOG educational objectives. This book provides those who are learning new skills to gain from experts' knowledge and experience. The associated course allows those in training to gain technical and non-technical skills, using simulation, in a safe environment and will ultimately improve the care offered to women.

Dr Clare McKenzie
RCOG Vice President (Education)

This book is intended for trainees attending the RCOG Operative Birth Simulation Training (ROBuST) course. However I anticipate that all obstetricians and obstetric trainees will find it useful and informative. To get the most out of the ROBuST course I recommend reading this book prior to attending but many of the chapters will also be useful for future reference. While this book covers the fundamentals of operative vaginal birth (OVB) it has been written to comprehensively cover the subject.

The individual chapters have been commissioned from nationally and internationally recognised experts, who have provided accounts of their own experiences and techniques. These techniques and alternatives will be taught on the hands-on ROBuST course.

This text and course have been developed to improve training in OVB worldwide, with the ultimate aim of improving safety for mothers and babies. Simulation training in obstetrics has the benefit of facilitating learning in technical and nontechnical skills in a safe environment, without any risk of patient harm.

The course is delivered in 1 day. It includes short lectures, demonstrations of technique (nonrotational and rotational OVB and caesarean section at full dilatation) and hands-on practice. Important generic skills including teamwork, communication and documentation are also covered.

I hope that you find this book useful and enjoy the course.

Alison Gale
Lead Editor and Simulation Advisor to RCOG

Chapter 1

Operative vaginal birth in the 21st century: a global perspective

Glen Mola

Key learning points

- The varied epidemiology of birthing around the world (and even the differences within one country) are attributable to both obstetric and midwifery practice styles and birthing agenda priorities.

- The skills required for vacuum extraction and forceps do have some commonality, but also have some quite distinct differences. Trainees wishing to master vacuum extraction skills for rotational and midcavity procedures need to pay careful attention to flexion point cup application. Vacuum extraction is truly an assisted birth strategy that requires coordination of strong uterine contractions, good maternal expulsive efforts and a combination of midwifery and obstetric skilled assistance during the procedure.

- Trainees who wish to gain additional operative obstetric experience in a developing country setting should choose training sites where the rate of operative vaginal birth (OVB) is more than 3%.

Historical perspectives

Obstetric forceps to assist birth of the baby date from the 16th century and were developed by three generations of the Chamberlen family. Between 1600 and 1920 over 700 types of forceps were designed; examples of about 100 of these can be viewed in the RCOG museum. Nowadays only four or five types of obstetric forceps are still in use. In most parts of the world, the proportion of assisted births performed by forceps is being overtaken by vacuum extraction procedures.

The earliest vaginal operations performed to assist birth were destructive. Destructive procedures to assist the birth of hydrocephalic and dead infants became standardised in the 19th century, only to become virtually obsolete in the 21st century in developed countries. Nevertheless, destructive operations are still life-saving procedures in developing countries, where performing caesarean section for neglected obstructed labour with a dead fetus can lead to maternal death, and delivering a hydrocephalic fetus by caesarean section is pointless if there is no expert paediatric neurosurgical and lifelong aftercare capacity available.

Although there were various attempts to design a vacuum extractor before the 1950s, modern vacuum extraction dates from 1953 when Professor Tage Malmström of Sweden developed the first modern vacuum extractor. Dr GC Bird made important modifications in the 1970s. In particular, Bird separated the suction and traction ports to make cup detachments less likely and also designed an occipito-posterior 'OP cup' with the suction port sited at the lateral margin of the cup, which allowed easier placement of the cup over the flexion point on the fetal scalp for occiput transverse and posterior positions.

In many ways OVB is at a crossroads: on the one hand rising caesarean section rates will be seen by some as making OVB virtually a redundant procedure, while in other places where OVB is practised, the clinical scene (both service and skill transfer capacity) can be quite disparate from country to country and even between facilities in the same country. Because of this, in many places, a full range of OVB skills have been lost or remain only in the hands of older practitioners who are no longer involved in teaching trainees. Nevertheless, there is still a window of opportunity for OVB skills to be retained; indeed, this is one of the reasons this book was commissioned by the RCOG.

Nowadays, concerns regarding OVB that need to be addressed at a national and institutional level in many countries are:

- what place does OVB have when second-stage problems arise?
- where should OVB be carried out?
- who should be authorised to perform it, and under what circumstances?

Current trends

General notes on vacuum extraction and forceps to assist vaginal birth

The RCOG Green-top Guideline No. 26: *Operative Vaginal Delivery* states that 'the operator should choose the instrument most appropriate to the clinical circumstances and their level of skill', and that 'obstetricians should be confident and competent in the use of both instruments for non-rotational deliveries and at least one instrument for rotational delivery'.[1] In fact this competency goal is quite difficult for most trainees to achieve in contemporary specialist training programmes. Many trainees complete their training within one obstetric service. In a particular hospital it is most unusual for there to be equal skill among the consultant trainers for both methods of assisted birth. Those obstetricians who mainly use forceps to assist birth sometimes consider using the vacuum extractor when there would be difficulty in applying the forceps, e.g. when the cervix is not fully dilated, when the head is in the midcavity or for rotational deliveries. It is not reasonable to expect good results when one uses an instrument that is not one's preferred instrument for more challenging clinical scenarios. On the other hand, vacuum extractions tend to be carried out by the more junior medical staff, and often without expert back-up from senior consultants who (for historical reasons) are more likely to be 'forceps users'.

The skills required for vacuum extraction and forceps do have some commonality, but distinctions can be made. However, the technique of use, good clinical practice points, common difficulties and pitfalls encountered and potential complications for the two procedures are markedly different.

The varying circumstances of practice between countries and hospitals within countries mean that, unless a trainee has opportunities to be trained in a variety of hospitals and regions, it is unlikely that the goals of the RCOG Green-top Guideline on operative vaginal delivery will be attained. One of the purposes of this book, and the ROBuST training course that accompanies it, is to ensure that trainees have the opportunity to develop skills in both methods of OVB.

Recent trends and perspectives in the developed world

Whereas UK caesarean section rates soared from 3% in 1960 to 33% in 2009 (since when the rate has remained steady),[2] in the USA and UK OVB rates have been quite steady since the 1970s at 9–12%.[2] However, in spite of fairly steady rates of assisted birth, the indications and clinical scenarios have changed considerably since the 1960s. Nowadays, few midcavity and 'trial' procedures are performed. Also, the trend to resort to caesarean section when there is malposition of the occiput or deflexion started before there was general availability of the Bird posterior cup, and before the development of other manoeuvrable cups such as the Kiwi Omnicup. The great majority of assisted births nowadays are what used to be called 'lift-outs'; i.e. from very low station and when the main problem is soft tissue resistance and inability of the woman to produce effective expulsive efforts to complete her delivery (often compounded by epidural analgesia).

From the 1950s (when the modern vacuum extractor was developed in Sweden by Malmström) and the 1970s, it was usual that hospitals, obstetric services and, indeed, countries were wont to use one method of assisted birth or the other, but not both. Even today it is not uncommon for hospitals to have 'rules' governing when trainees may or may not assist vaginal birth; indeed, the forceps (or certain types of forceps) or the vacuum extractor have been banned from some obstetric services. This has usually followed a complication caused by improper use of a particular instrument.

Although there have been attempts since the 1990s in most developed country obstetric services to train and use both methods of assisted birth, two other distinct trends have developed:

- where both instruments are used, there is a steady trend for a greater proportion of the OVB procedures to be performed using the vacuum extractor[3]
- in many places fewer vaginal births are assisted and caesarean section is being employed more often for second-stage problems.[4]

As a result of these trends, young obstetricians may begin specialist practice with little experience in performing midcavity or rotational procedures. The trend to subspecialisation has also contributed to de-skilling in operative obstetrics as many newly qualified consultants regard their obstetric practice as only a transitional career phase.

Trends in the developing world

In the developing world, tradition and local conventions often reign supreme and the hierarchical nature of the medical profession make it difficult for someone to (re-)introduce skills. In large capital city teaching hospitals there may be only four or five consultants in a clinical unit or practice and, for all sorts of reasons, both logistic and socioprofessional, there is often little in the way of hands-on teaching for trainees in the labour ward. Lack of hands-on supervision in the labour ward can mean that there is a trend to use caesarean section as the 'solution' for every difficulty in labour. Some obstetric services in Africa and the Middle East have caesarean section rates that rival the developed world but OVB rates of less than 1%.[5] Asian countries have more varied practice and trends[6] (Table 1.1).

In the developing world, the problem of low public practice salaries means that most specialists survive on private practice income; however, it is difficult to run a successful private practice and at the same time be available to provide hands-on assistance for public hospital emergencies. Consequently, trainees often find themselves having to work things out for themselves: OVB is not a skill that is easy to work out by yourself. Therefore, after a couple of generations of little hands-on skills training in the labour ward, young obstetricians begin specialist practice with little training or experience in assisted birth and are therefore unable to instruct the next generation of trainees in this skill.

The Dr GC Bird legacy and the Papua New Guinea experience

GC Bird trained in the UK and practiced obstetrics mostly in Kenya and Papua New Guinea. From 1968 to 1980, Dr Bird was Director of Obstetrics at the Port Moresby General Hospital in Papua New Guinea. In the early 1970s, he was involved in the first multicentre observational trials and graphing of cervical dilatation that led to the development of the partograph for the modern management of labour. During this period, Dr Bird became interested in the mechanics of assisted birth – he was one of the first to understand the importance of a flexing application of the vacuum cup to minimise failure with vacuum extraction.

Up to the 1960s, OVB was often employed to overcome minor degrees of cephalopelvic disproportion. With the forceps it is possible to exert quite extreme amounts of traction force: when this is excessive it is not uncommon that the infant sustains some birth trauma. The vacuum extractor, on the other hand, tends to detach when excessive traction force is applied. However, in the clinical scenario when there is 'tightness of fit' of the head in the pelvis, the vacuum extractor itself does not occupy any space in the pelvis, and by its first action in optimising flexion and correcting asynclitism it can overcome minor degrees of apparent disproportion without causing damage to either the woman or her baby.

Table 1.1 Comparison of differences in fertility, resource capacity and social issues that make the threshold for caesarean section low and spontaneous vaginal birth and operative vaginal birth more difficult to achieve between developing and developed countries

Issue	Developed country practice	Developing country practice
Total fertility rate	Low: most women have a desired family size of ~2	High: many women desire 4+ children
Client attitudes	Clients and families feel that they should be able to make decisions about obstetric care	Clients and families come to health professionals because they feel that they know what is best
Resources: human, equipment, drugs, logistics	Rarely do resource constraints impact on quality of midwifery care and obstetrical decision making	Midwifery care is often challenged and medical care needs to take resource constraints into account
Medico-legal factors	Perinatal factors commonly the subject of litigation if an outcome is not optimal	Most patients would not think of suing health staff as long as they considered that staff tried their best in the circumstances
Midwifery and support person views	Sometimes women are encouraged to not consider interventions even when a minor intervention early on could keep labour on a 'normal' track – leading to situations where a woman feels that CS is now the only 'reasonable option'	Midwives encourage women to believe that they can achieve a normal birth, but are happy to resort to sensible intervention when this would be beneficial
Society views	CS is as 'normal' as spontaneous birth or OVB	CS should only be performed if a woman cannot give birth to her baby safely: OVB is considered assistance to normal birth and not an 'operation'
Access to theatre and anaesthesia and blood, etc.	Available within the hour	May not be available at all or only after extended delay

CS = caesarean section; OVB = operative vaginal birth.

6

Papua New Guinea, common to developing countries, has many remote villages where referral is difficult or impossible. For this reason it is logistically not possible for a woman to be referred to hospital when there is prolonged labour, and a caesarean scar may be a morbid handicap in subsequent pregnancies when there may be no access to antenatal or intrapartum care. For these reasons, the Papua New Guinea obstetric service has maintained a focus on effective vacuum extraction and keeping the caesarean section rate at around 5%. Over the past 40 years the rate of vacuum extraction failure at Port Moresby General Hospital has been steady at about 2.5%.[7]

OVB in low-resource countries

In the typical developing country labour ward where OVB is not commonly performed

In Asia, assisted birth rates are mostly less than 5%,[6] and in Africa and South America the rates in big city hospitals are mostly only 1–2%.[8,9] Concomitantly, caesarean rates are as high (or higher) than in developed countries, sometimes with devastating consequences both contemporaneously (because of operative and anaesthetic risks) and in the longer term because of the scar in the uterus and the risks in the next pregnancy.

The only time that assisted birth is performed in these circumstances is when the head is on the perineum and the woman is unable to push it out despite an episiotomy being performed. In the 1990s there was a spate of papers published that lamented the loss of this obstetric skill;[10] however, by and large the situation has not changed much.

Where operative vaginal birth is routinely performed when it is the best option to expedite birth

There are parts of the developing world where OVB is performed as a reasonable alternative to prolonged expulsive efforts and caesarean section. It is often in church agency and rural district hospitals that OVB skills have been maintained, as well as some national sites (e.g. Port Moresby General Hospital), which have now become centres of excellence for OVB skills. There are other places such as Cambodia that have seriously taken on the World Health Organization (WHO) view that assisted vaginal birth is a 'comprehensive emergency obstetric care function'[11,12] and have made a national effort to improve and roll out training in OVB.

In the developing world caesarean section can be quite dangerous for the woman not only in the current pregnancy because of surgical and anaesthetic difficulties, but also in subsequent pregnancies owing to the scar in her uterus, particularly if she is not assured of being able to access antenatal, labour and postnatal care in the next pregnancy (Table 1.2).

In the developing countries where operative obstetric skills have been maintained, operative vaginal birth is often carried out when there are concerns in terms of 'fit' (i.e. relative cephalopelvic disproportion). In these circumstances, unless there is a contraindication, labour is augmented when there is delay in the first (and second) stages and OVB will subsequently take place in the presence of caput and considerable moulding of the head. Epidural analgesia is mostly not available in developing countries. Moreover, there is a common view (both in the community and among maternity care professionals) that women are expected to 'push out their baby'. Under these circumstances practitioners make a concerted effort to avoid vacuum extraction failure by:

- augmenting contractions to maximise the three to four expulsive efforts of the procedure
- enlisting a midwife to encourage the woman to maximise her expulsive efforts for each of the tractions (and, in the author's opinion, sometimes exerting some fundal pressure with these efforts as well, when this is an acceptable part of intrapartum care – this would not be acceptable practice in the UK)
- the operator exerting as much traction as is safe to do.

In a trial situation, symphysiotomy may be used to complete OVB if the trial does not lead to satisfactory progress with the first several tractions.

In short, to minimise vacuum extraction failure and risk of scalp trauma, the message should be to maximise 'push' and minimise 'pull'.

Training and skill attainment for OVB

Historical training models and their advantages and disadvantages

Up to the 1970s it was common in many parts of the world for preservice trainees to be shown how to perform OVB as an 'elective' procedure, i.e. when the procedure was not fully indicated for clinical reasons, but for 'training purposes'. This style of training had the advantage of helping all trainees to

Table 1.2 Comparison between developed and developing countries in terms of the risks and benefits of caesarean section and vaginal birth (including operative vaginal birth)

Caesarean section risk issues	Developed countries	Developing countries
TFR Each birth increases the risk for a woman with a CS scar	TFR is commonly about 2	TFR is often 4+
Repeat CS	Elective repeat CS is often performed	Women will usually undergo trial of scar
Risk of placenta previa and abnormal placentation	Can be handled in most cases without serious morbidity or mortality risk	Placenta previa can be a life-threatening condition, and abnormal placentation has a very high mortality rate
Operative risks	Expertise is adequate and referral to more experienced practitioners for complications routine	Surgery may be performed by nonspecialists with limited experience, and there my be no access to experienced practitioners when complications develop
Anaesthetic and blood transfusion capacity	Anaesthetic expertise and adequate supplies of blood routinely available	Neither obstetrical anaesthetic expertise nor blood availability is routinely adequate
CS rates increase to high levels	Not a big problem	Can have a significant impact on the maternal mortality rate
Risks for subsequent pregnancies	Not commonly significant; only if abnormal placentation develops	If a woman cannot be assured of antenatal, and intrapartum care in the next pregnancy, a CS scar could be a 'death sentence'
Community expectations	CS is a expected to be performed for every difficulty in labour	Most women and families expect women to give birth vaginally unless there is a serious problem

CS = caesarean section; OVB = operative vaginal birth; TFR = total fertility rate.

become familiar with procedures; however, it suffers from the obvious disadvantage that the patient became a training 'resource', often without appropriate consent.

In the 1970s the 'see one, do one, teach one' mantra became a popular clinical training model. With complex procedures such as OVB, this can lead to poor outcomes and inadequate skill transfer. Bad habits formed in the 'do one' phase can also lead to passing on wrong messages in the 'teach one' phase.

A better model for OVB training might be termed the coaching model. This model starts with theoretical knowledge, moves on to observed clinical practice, then simulated practice on mannequins, and finally to direct supervision by the trainer in the clinical area. In fact, this is what is envisaged in the ROBuST training programme.

Skills training workshops, mannequins and on the job training

Nowadays clinical skills workshops abound. There are skills training workshops available in ultrasound diagnosis, operative pelvic and laparoscopic surgery, colposcopy and other gynaecological procedures; skills training workshops in emergency and newborn care are many and varied too.

Recently, various mannequins have been produced to assist with emergency obstetric care skills training; these have differing merits and vary in terms of fidelity and resilience.

Sau et al.[13] asked the question 'Vacuum extraction: is there any need to improve the current training in the UK?' and, from the results of their paper, clearly the answer was a resounding 'yes'. Now is the time to put this into evidence-based practice.

References

1. Royal College of Obstetricians and Gynaecologists. *Operative vaginal delivery*. Green-top Guideline No. 26. London: RCOG; 2011.

2. Hamilton BE, Martin JA, Ventura SJ. Births: preliminary data for 2010. *Natl Vital Stat Rep* 2011;60:1–25.

3. Miksovsky P, Watson WJ. Obstetric vacuum extraction: state of the art in the new millennium, *Obstet Gynecol Surv* 2001;56:11.

4. Menacker F, Martin JA. BirthStats: rates of cesarean delivery, and unassisted and assisted vaginal delivery, United States, 1996, 2000, and 2006. *Birth* 2009;36:167.

5. Van Roosmalen J. From audit of perinatal deaths to recommendations for management of dystocia. Presentation made at the Colloquium on the management of difficult labour problems, University of Durban Department of Obstetrics, 2002.

6. Lumbiganon P, Laopaiboon M, Gülmezoglu AM, Souza JP, Taneepanichskul S, Ruyan P, et al.; WHO global survey research group on maternal and perinatal health. Method of delivery and pregnancy outcomes in Asia: the WHO survey on maternal and perinatal health 2007–2008. *Lancet* 2010;375:490–9.

7. Mola GDL, Kuk J. Operative vaginal delivery at Port Moresby General Hospital from 1977–2010. *PNG Med J* 2011;54:174–84.

8. Villar J, Valladares E, Wojdyla D, Zavaleta N, Carroli G, Velazco A, et al. Caesarean delivery rates and pregnancy outcomes; the 2005 global survey on maternal and perinatal health in South America. *Lancet* 2006;367:1819–29.

9. Shah A, Fawole B, M'imunya JM, Amokrane F, Nafiou I, Wolomby JJ, et al. Caesarean delivery outcomes from the WHO global survey on maternal and perinatal health in Africa. *Int J Gynaecol Obstet* 2009;107:191–7.

10. Bailey PE. Disappearing rates of assisted vaginal delivery: time to reverse the trend. *Int J Gynaecol Obstet* 2005;91:89–96.

11. UNICEF, WHO, *UNFPA. Guidelines for monitoring the availability and use of obstetric services*. New York: UNICEF; 1997.

12. Paxton A, Maine D, Freddman L, Fry D, Lobis S. The evidence for emergency obstetric care. *Int J Gynaecol Obstet* 2005;88:181–93.

13. Sau A, Sau M, Ahmed H, Brown R. Vacuum extraction: is there any need to improve the current training in the UK? *Acta Obstet Gynecol Scand* 2004;83:466–70.

Chapter 2
Indications and assessment for operative vaginal birth

Deirdre Murphy and Meenakshi Ramphul

Key learning points

- Operative vaginal birth (OVB) should be offered only when the benefits outweigh the potential risks, taking account of both maternal and neonatal perspectives.
- A systematic clinical assessment, effective communication and expertise in the intended procedure are prerequisites for OVB.
- The position and station of the fetal head are important indicators of the level of skill required of the operator and will also impact on the choice of instrument and where the birth is conducted (labour room versus operating theatre).

The decision whether or not to perform an OVB is a complex one. Choosing the most appropriate mode of birth, conducted under optimal circumstances, in the most appropriate place, by a competent operator, are the main elements for safe birth of a healthy infant while maintaining a positive experience for the mother and her partner. The risk of maternal and neonatal morbidity is increased with OVBs, although with careful practice these risks are low.[1] Close attention needs to be paid to the indication for OVB and to clinical assessment before any attempt at the chosen procedure.

There are two alternatives to OVB. The first, continued pushing aiming for a spontaneous vaginal birth, may be unwise if there is evidence of fetal compromise or diminished maternal reserve. The second, a caesarean section at full dilatation, is a complex intervention associated with increased risks of maternal morbidity (major haemorrhage, extended hospital stay) and neonatal morbidity (higher rates of admission to the neonatal unit).[2] Overall, women who have vaginal births (albeit with assistance) tend to be more satisfied with the birth than those who have emergency caesarean sections.[3] The risk of intrapartum complications in subsequent pregnancies is greatly reduced if a safe OVB can be completed.[4]

Classification of Operative Vaginal Birth

OVBs are classified primarily by the station and position of the fetal head (Table 2.1). The station of the fetal head refers to descent of the leading part of the skull within the birth canal in relation to the maternal ischial spines.[5] The position refers to the orientation of the fetal occiput (in a vertex presentation) in relation to the maternal pubic symphysis. The fetal station must be at the level of the ischial spines (station 0) or below to fulfil the criteria for safe OVB. In most circumstances this correlates with zero-fifths of the fetal head palpable abdominally (a deeply engaged presenting part). The exception is with a deflexed OP position at the level of the ischial spines, where there may be up to (but no more than) one-fifth of the fetal head palpable abdominally for the classification to be considered midcavity and therefore potentially suitable for OVB. Occipito-anterior (OA) positions are less challenging for OVB than occipito-transverse (OT) or occipito-posterior (OP) positions (fetal malpositions requiring rotation). OVBs are further subclassified into those that require or do not require rotation.

A standard classification should be used to enable clear communication, benchmarking, audit and comparisons between studies. The RCOG uses adapted criteria from the guideline of the American College of Obstetricians and Gynecologists (ACOG)[6,7] (Table 2.1). The first important stage in training obstetricians for OVB is to ensure consistency and accuracy in assessment of the station and position of the fetal head and therefore in classification of the planned birth. The supervising obstetrician should be confident that this competency has been achieved before indirect supervision is provided.

Indications

Operative vaginal births are performed when birth needs to be expedited and may be indicated for conditions of the fetus or the mother or both (Table 2.2). The overall premise should be to offer OVB when the benefits outweigh the risks.

Table 2.1 Classification for operative vaginal delivery

Outlet	Fetal scalp visible without separating labia
	Fetal skull has reached the pelvic floor
	Sagittal suture is in the anterio-posterior diameter or right or left occiputo-anterior or -posterior position (rotation does not exceed 45°)
	Fetal head is at or on the perineum
Low	Leading point of the skull (not caput) is at station plus 2 cm or more and not on the pelvic floor
	Two subdivisions:
	■ rotation of ≤45° from the occipito-anterior position
	■ rotation of >45° including the occipito-posterior position
Mid	Fetal head is no more than one-fifth palpable per abdomen
	Leading point of the skull is above station plus 2 cm but not above ischial spines
	Two subdivisions:
	■ rotation of ≤45° from the occipito-anterior position
	■ rotation of >45° including the occipito-posterior position
High	Not included in the classification as operative vaginal delivery is not recommended in this situation where the head is two-fifths or more palpable abdominally and the presenting part is above the level of the ischial spines

Adapted from the Royal College of Obstetricians and Gynaecologists 2011.[6]

The most common indication for OVB is inadequate progress in the second stage of labour. In nulliparous women, a delay in the second stage with regional anaesthesia is diagnosed when birth is not imminent after 3 hours from the diagnosis of full cervical dilatation (total passive and active second stage) or after 2 hours without regional anaesthesia.[8] In multiparous women, this is diagnosed when birth is not imminent after 2 hours with regional anaesthesia (total passive and active second stage) or 1 hour without regional anaesthesia.[8] It should be noted that where a woman has been pushing effectively for 30–40 minutes with no discernible progress, earlier assessment may be appropriate as a fetal malposition, malpresentation or cephalopelvic disproportion may be present. In these circumstances a senior assessment should be sought with regard to ongoing management, rather than persisting with 2 hours of unproductive pushing that may exacerbate the problem.

Table 2.2 Indications and contraindications for OVB

Type	Indication (relative)	Contraindication (relative)	Instrument-specific contraindication
Inadequate progress	Nulliparous: lack of continuing progress for 3 hours* with regional anaesthesia or 2 hours* without regional anaesthesia Multiparous: lack of continuing progress for 2 hours* with regional anaesthesia or 1 hour* without regional anaesthesia	Suspected cephalopelvic disproportion	
Fetal	Presumed fetal compromise	Predisposition to fracture (e.g. osteogenesis imperfecta) Malpresentation (brow, face mento-posterior)	**Vacuum:** Gestation <34–36 weeks Face presentation Fetal bleeding disorders **Midcavity/ rotational forceps:** Fetal bleeding disorders
Maternal	Fatigue/exhaustion Medical conditions that preclude maternal effort such as cardiac disease, hypertensive crisis, cerebrovascular disease	Refusal to consent	

* Total of active and passive second stage of labour.

15

Suspected fetal compromise, as revealed by a suspicious or pathological fetal heart rate pattern on cardiotocography (CTG), is also a common indication for OVB. Special circumstances include suspected sepsis (maternal pyrexia, maternal tachycardia, fetal tachycardia, foul-smelling amniotic fluid), fetal growth restriction, preterm labour, intrapartum vaginal bleeding, previous caesarean section and fetal heart rate abnormalities in a second twin. In these circumstances the fetal reserve may be diminished and the decision to intervene should take into account the potential for a more rapidly deteriorating acid–base status in the fetus.

Maternal conditions that indicate OVB are most commonly maternal distress or fatigue. Less common medical conditions that preclude prolonged maternal effort include maternal cardiac disease, hypertensive crisis, cerebrovascular disease or respiratory compromise.

Most indications are relative and there may be more than one indication to perform an OVB, for example in cases where there is maternal fatigue with suspected fetal compromise after 1 hour of pushing. When to intervene is therefore a balance of risks and benefits and will depend on individual clinical circumstances and maternal preferences.

Contraindications

Operative vaginal birth is contraindicated when the cervix is less than fully dilated and when the fetal head is not deeply engaged (station above the ischial spines and/or more than one-fifth of the fetal head palpable abdominally) (Table 2.3). Operative vaginal birth is relatively contraindicated in cases of fetal bleeding disorders (e.g. suspected thrombocytopenia) or a predisposition to fracture (e.g. osteogenesis imperfecta) (Table 2.2). However, in some circumstances it may be more traumatic for the fetus to be born by CS, for example in advanced labour with the fetal head deep in the pelvis. In cases of blood-borne viral infections such as hepatitis B/C and HIV, OVB is not contraindicated but, as there is an increased risk of fetal abrasion or scalp trauma, it is sensible to avoid potentially difficult midcavity or rotational procedures.

Forceps can be used for some malpresentations such as face presentation in a mento-anterior position or for the after-coming head of a breech. In cases of brow or a mento-posterior face presentation, instrumental delivery should not be attempted unless the brow can be flexed to a vertex presentation or deflexed to a face presentation and the mento-posterior face presentation requires rotation to mento-anterior which can be achieved manually. These procedures require specialist expertise and are not suitable for novice practitioners.

Table 2.3 Prerequisites for operative vaginal delivery*

Full abdominal and vaginal examination	■ Head is no more than one-fifth palpable per abdomen
	■ Station at spines or below
	■ Cervix is fully dilated and membranes ruptured
	■ Diagnosis of the exact fetal head position (to ensure proper placement of instrument)
	■ Assessment of caput and moulding (irreducible moulding may indicate cephalopelvic disproportion)
	■ Pelvis is deemed adequate
Preparation of mother	■ Clear explanation should be given and informed consent obtained
	■ Appropriate anaesthesia
	■ Maternal bladder should be emptied; indwelling catheter should be removed or balloon deflated
	■ Aseptic technique
Preparation of staff	■ Operator should have knowledge, experience and skill necessary
	■ Adequate facilities are available (appropriate equipment, bed, lighting)
	■ Back-up plan in place in case of failure of OVB. When conducting midcavity births, theatre staff should be immediately available to allow a caesarean section to be performed without delay (<30 minutes). A senior obstetrician competent in performing midcavity OVBs should be present if a junior trainee is performing the birth
	■ Anticipation of complications that may arise (e.g. shoulder dystocia, postpartum haemorrhage)
	■ Personnel present that are trained in neonatal resuscitation

* Adapted from the Royal College of Obstetricians and Gynaecologists 2011.[6]

Vacuum-assisted births are contraindicated when the gestation is less than 34 completed weeks as there is a risk of cephalhaematoma, intracranial haemorrhage, subgaleal haemorrhage and neonatal jaundice. It has also been suggested that the vacuum extractor should be avoided at less than 36 completed weeks of gestation because of the risk of subgaleal and intracranial haemorrhage. However, there is insufficient evidence to establish the safety of the vacuum extractor at gestations between 34 and 36 weeks. As a general rule, most obstetricians avoid vacuum-assisted birth at gestations less than 36 completed weeks.

Maternal consent is a prerequisite for OVB; therefore, refusal to consent to OVB is a contraindication. However, the alternatives and associated risks must be clearly outlined to the woman and her partner. Prolonged pushing may be detrimental to the fetus, particularly in cases of suspected fetal compromise or uncertain fetal reserve. The woman needs to be aware that there is increased maternal and neonatal morbidity associated with caesarean section at full dilatation when performed with the head low in the pelvis and this may be more traumatic than an OVB.[2] Ideally, these discussions should take place in the antenatal period, or earlier in the course of the labour if limitations have been expressed in the birth plan. A similar approach is required where a woman has stated a preference for a particular choice of instrument.

Prerequisites

Before performing an OVB, a careful assessment of the clinical situation, clear communication with the mother, partner and healthcare personnel and expertise in the planned procedure are essential (Table 2.3).

The indication for the procedure should be established and clearly documented. Informed consent should be obtained from the woman after explicit counselling regarding the indication, advantages and disadvantages and nature of the procedure. This may be difficult to achieve in what is essentially an emergency setting, but information should be given to the woman between contractions and, where possible, the birth plan of the mother should be taken into account and discussed. The principles of obtaining valid consent in labour should be followed and consent advice from the RCOG on OVB should be followed.[6]

The alternatives to OVB, i.e. continued pushing or caesarean section, should also be discussed with the woman, outlining the advantages and disadvantages of each option. For OVBs in the labour room, verbal consent should be obtained and clearly documented in the notes, with an endeavour to obtain written consent when possible. However, for OVBs in theatre, written consent should be obtained.[6]

A systematic abdominal and vaginal examination should be performed to establish the size of the fetus, engagement, position, station and attitude of the fetal head, the pelvic dimensions and the adequacy of analgesia, as outlined below. For low or outlet births, infiltration of local anaesthetic into the perineum may suffice, but a pudendal block may be required. For midcavity births, especially rotational procedures, regional anaesthesia (epidural or spinal) is optimal. Before the procedure, the bladder should be emptied by 'in and out' catheterisation to reduce the risk of urethral or bladder damage. If an indwelling catheter is in place, the bulb should be deflated.

The operator should have the appropriate knowledge, skills and experience required. Trainees should be adequately supervised by more senior obstetricians, especially in cases of midcavity or rotational births. Operative vaginal births can be associated with maternal and fetal morbidity, particularly in cases of sequential use of instruments (vacuum followed by forceps) and failed OVBs (vacuum and/or forceps followed by caesarean section), which are often related to inexperience of the operator.[2,9]

Assessment before Operative Vaginal Birth

General considerations

An open and positive first impression is important in building rapport and trust with the woman and her carers. The obstetrician should attempt to gauge the atmosphere and morale within the room and respond sensitively and with empathy to the woman's situation. Birth partners will sometimes advocate on behalf of the woman but care should be taken especially if there are communication difficulties. A professionally trained interpreter should be used wherever possible for women who speak a different language or who are hearing impaired.

Clinical history to date

Before attempting an OVB, it is important to review the woman's medical and antenatal history carefully to exclude any contraindications to OVB and to anticipate any potential complications (e.g. cephalopelvic disproportion, shoulder dystocia, neonatal injury or postpartum haemorrhage). The past obstetric history, presence of diabetes, antenatal diagnosis of fetal concerns (abnormal growth, oligohydramnios, abnormal fetal Doppler studies, fetal anomaly) and maternal blood results (serology, anaemia, rhesus) may be of particular relevance. The partogram should be assessed looking at progress in the first stage of labour, efficiency of uterine contractions and the use of oxytocin. The maternal body mass index, vital signs and hydration status should be noted. Particular attention should be paid to a maternal pyrexia or tachycardia, hypertension or haematuria.

Review of the fetal status

The fetal status should be assessed as a matter of priority as this will determine the need for urgency in terms of intervention. Women identified as high risk antenatally or in labour should be offered continuous electronic fetal monitoring (EFM) with cardiotocography (CTG) (Table 2.4). The four features of the fetal heart recording (baseline fetal heart rate, variability, accelerations, decelerations) and the uterine contractions (care should be taken to record uterine activity adequately) should be noted to classify the trace as normal, suspicious or pathological.[8] Any fetal blood samples (FBS) taken in the first or second stage of labour should also be noted. Meconium-stained liquor should be considered a possible sign of fetal compromise, although this may be a normal finding in prolonged pregnancies. Absence of liquor should also be considered abnormal and may reflect undetected placental insufficiency. A degree of urgency is required for CTGs that are classified as pathological and for fetal blood samples with pH below 7.20.[8]

Abdominal examination

A systematic abdominal examination using Leopold's four manoeuvres should be undertaken. The fetal lie and presentation should be confirmed and the fetal size should be assessed clinically. A small-for-gestational-age fetus is an important finding in terms of potential diminished fetal reserve in labour and also ease of delivery. A clinically large fetus may be associated with cephalopelvic disproportion and failed instrumental delivery or with shoulder dystocia and subsequent postpartum haemorrhage. Engagement of the fetal head occurs when the widest transverse diameter of the fetal head (biparietal diameter [BPD]) passes through the pelvic inlet.[5] Engagement of the fetal head should be ascertained abdominally and is described in terms of 'fifths' palpable, depending on how much of the head is palpable abdominally. Operative vaginal births should be attempted only where no more than one-fifth of the head is palpable abdominally and in the majority of cases

Table 2.4 Maternal and fetal factors where electronic fetal monitoring is recommended[8]

Maternal	Fetal
Pre-eclampsia	Fetal growth restriction
Diabetes	Prematurity (gestation <37 weeks)
Prolonged rupture of membranes	Meconium-stained liquor
>24 hours	Abnormal Doppler artery velocimetry
Previous caesarean section	Oligohydramnios
Antepartum haemorrhage or vaginal	Breech presentation
bleeding in labour	Multiple pregnancies
Induced labour	
Prolonged pregnancy (>42 weeks)	
Maternal pyrexia	
Epidural analgesia	
Oxytocin augmentation	
Maternal medical disorders	

there will be zero-fifths palpable abdominally. The position of the fetal back should also be sought to help define the position of the fetal head, although in practice this is often difficult.

Vaginal examination

A systematic vaginal examination should be performed to confirm full cervical dilatation, a cephalic vertex presentation, the position, station and attitude (degree of flexion) of the fetal head, the degree of caput (scalp swelling) and moulding (closure and overlap of the skull bones), and to form a subjective impression of the pelvic dimensions. In addition it is extremely helpful to assess whether rotation (if required) and descent occur during a contraction with active pushing.

Palpation of each fontanelle (anterior and posterior) and the suture lines of the fetal skull should be carried out to determine the fetal head position as accurately as possible (Figures 2.1 and 2.2). However, digital vaginal examination is not always accurate, especially in the presence of caput, moulding and asynclitism.[10,11] The accuracy of digital vaginal examination to determine the fetal head position in the second stage of labour has been compared with transabdominal ultrasound and reported to be between 35% and 80%.[10–18] The role of ultrasound to determine the fetal head position before OVBs has been investigated in two studies of

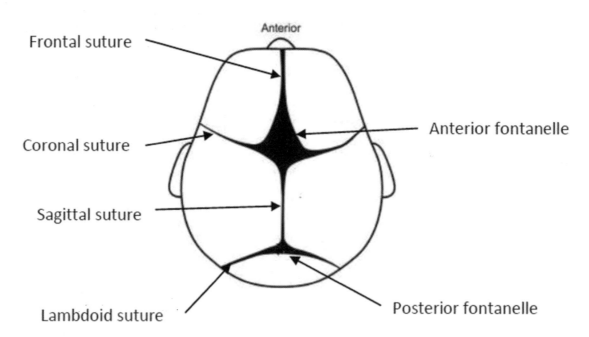

Figure 2.1 Landmarks of the fetal skull

64 and 50 women, respectively.[19,20] Digital vaginal examination was inaccurate in one-quarter of cases before OVB in one study.[19] In the other study, a midwife measured the distance between the centre of the chignon and the flexion point immediately after birth. In the group with digital examination and ultrasound assessment, the mean distance between the centre of the chignon and the flexion point was 2.1±1.3 cm compared with 2.8±1.0 cm in the group with digital examination alone, a small but statistically significant difference.[20] Although promising, current evidence is insufficient to support routine use of ultrasound as part of assessment prior to OVB.

The station of the fetal head should be ascertained routinely on vaginal examination. However, similar to the issues with inaccuracy of the fetal head position, there is evidence that vaginal assessment of the station of the fetal head is not always reliable.[21] Transabdominal and translabial ultrasound have been used in a research setting to assess station of the fetal head but are not used routinely in current practice.[22–24] Henrich et al.[25] evaluated the correlation between head descent as assessed on translabial ultrasound during active pushing and successful vacuum extraction. They assessed the widest fetal head diameter, fetal head movement (head descent) in terms of the 'infrapubic line' (an imaginary line perpendicular to the long axis of the symphysis pubis extending to the dorsal part of the pelvis) and the head direction with respect to the symphysis. The authors found that objective head descent demonstrated by infrapubic translabial ultrasound (ITU) below the infrapubic line and a 'head up' sign (head pointing ventrally) was a good

Direct occipito anterior

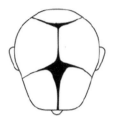

Right occipito anterior

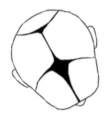

Left occipito anterior

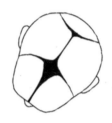

Right occipito transverse

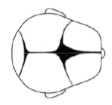

Left occipito transverse

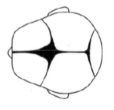

Right occipito posterior

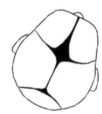

Left occipito posterior

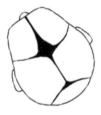

Direct occipito posterior

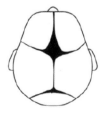

Figure 2.2 Fetal head position

prognostic factor for successful vacuum extraction (11 out of 20 cases), while no descent was associated with difficult or failed extraction.

Another tool investigated to improve the accuracy of assessment of the station of the fetal head is the StationMaster (a modified amniotomy hook that relocates the reference point for defining the station from the ischial spines to the posterior fourchette).[26] A simulation study of the StationMaster using a mannequin pelvis showed that it was more accurate than digital assessment of fetal head station.[26]

The position and station of the fetal head are important indicators of the level of skill required of the operator and will also have an impact on the choice of instrument and where the birth is carried out (labour room versus operating theatre). Rotation and descent of the presenting part with maternal effort during a contraction is a good prognostic factor for successful OVB but cases with minimal or no descent should be treated with caution. Similarly, the presence of marked caput or moulding of the fetal skull bones should be established, as irreducible moulding may be a warning sign for cephalopelvic disproportion.

Observation period

Observation of the maternal effort and the woman's psychological status during active pushing often helps the operator decide when to intervene and which instrument to use. The perspective of the woman and the midwife caring for her will assist the decision-making process. This may not be possible in cases of emergency such as fetal bradycardia.

Choice of instruments

The choice of forceps or vacuum extractor will depend on the clinical circumstances and on the operator's competencies and personal preferences. Forceps birth may be preferred in instances where there is diminished maternal effort (e.g. maternal exhaustion, dense epidural block, general anaesthesia), for preterm births (<34–36 weeks of gestation), for rotational births, after a failed attempt at vacuum extraction, for delivery of the after-coming head in breech births and for low-cavity births with suspected fetal coagulopathy or thrombocytopenia. A vacuum-assisted birth may be preferred where analgesia is limited, for low-cavity or outlet births and for rotational births in preference to manual rotation or rotational forceps. The relative merits of vacuum extraction and forceps have been explored in a Cochrane systematic review of randomised controlled trials and are summarised in Table 2.5.[27]

Table 2.5 Relative merits of vacuum extraction and forceps[27]

	Advantages	Disadvantages
Vacuum extractor	Less maternal perineal and vaginal trauma Less analgesia required	Cephalhaematoma more likely Retinal haemorrhage more likely Use of sequential instruments more likely
Forceps	Successful vaginal birth more likely with single instrument	Maternal perineal and vaginal trauma more likely Increased analgesia requirements Neonatal facial nerve palsy more likely

Forceps

There are over 700 types of forceps and there have been no randomised controlled trials comparing forceps types. The three main types (outlet, midcavity and rotational) can be used in specific situations but require differing levels of expertise.[28] Forceps are more likely to be successful at completing vaginal birth with a single instrument than vacuum.[29] Forceps are usually faster than vacuum extraction, which may be critical in cases of fetal bradycardia, cord prolapse or placental abruption.[30] However, compared with vacuum, forceps are associated with a higher risk of vaginal trauma, third- and fourth-degree tears, facial injuries to the neonate and increased analgesia requirements.[27] Rotational birth with Kiellands forceps carries additional potential risks and requires specific expertise and training. Manual rotation followed by direct traction forceps may be preferred depending on the operator's skills and experience.[6]

Vacuum

Vacuum cups can be metal, plastic or silicone. The vacuum extractor is being used increasingly as the instrument of first choice. This is likely to reflect the need for less analgesia/anaesthesia and the lower incidence of maternal pelvic floor trauma.[27] However, compared with forceps birth, vacuum extraction is associated with an increased risk of neonatal cephalhaematoma, retinal haemorrhage and maternal concern about wellbeing of the neonate.[27] A Cochrane systematic review showed that the metal cup was more likely than soft cups to result in a successful vaginal birth with no difference in maternal perineal trauma.[27] However, the metal cup was associated with an increased risk of neonatal bruising, cephalhaematoma and scalp injury.[27] Two randomised controlled trials comparing a disposible vacuum device (Kiwi OmniCup) with standard vacuum cups reported high rates of instrument failure requiring sequential use of forceps (20–30%) with a significantly higher incidence of failure with the disposible device.[31–32]

Operative vaginal birth in theatre

Operative vaginal births that are anticipated to have a higher rate of failure should be carried out in a place where immediate safe recourse to caesarean section can be undertaken.[6] Fetal hypoxic-ischaemic injuries have been attributed to delay between a failed OVB and a caesarean section. Failure rates are higher for midcavity births, women with a high body mass index (BMI) (>30 kg/m^2), babies with a birthweight over 4000 g and malpositions of the fetal head, in particular the OP position.

Transfer to theatre for an OVB with preparations in case of a caesarean section has the advantages of facilitating optimal anaesthesia, enhanced clinical assessment and, where appropriate hospital protocols are in place, senior support for the birth. There will be a delay in the decision-to-delivery interval (DDI) associated with transferring a woman to theatre compared with giving birth in the labour room, but this has not been found to be associated with adverse neonatal outcomes.[33] The decision to transfer the woman to theatre should balance the benefits in terms of safety should OVB fail, with the potential negatives in terms of delay in the DDI and the additional anxiety for the woman and her partner.

Complications

Complications are inevitable to some degree with any operative procedure. Appropriate use of OVB by well-trained obstetricians should minimise the risk of complications and alleviate the risks to the mother and baby of delaying birth. However, failure to assess the clinical scenario correctly can lead to significant maternal and neonatal morbidity. Failure to diagnose a fetal malposition increases the likelihood of failed OVB, with the additional morbidity of sequential use of instruments or second-stage caesarean section. Misjudging the fetal size or ignoring signs of cephalopelvic disproportion may lead to failed OVB or shoulder dystocia. When assessing fetal wellbeing, signs of sepsis or significant CTG abnormalities may be missed with delayed birth resulting in neonatal hypoxic-ischaemic encephalopathy and subsequent cerebral palsy.[2,9,29,34]

Poorly conducted OVBs are associated with an increased incidence of third- and fourth-degree tears, vaginal wall and cervical lacerations, postpartum haemorrhage, long-term pelvic floor sequelae and psychological distress. For the neonate they are associated with traumatic injuries, hypoxic-ischaemic encephalopathy, cerebral haemorrhage and, rarely, perinatal death. Caesarean section in the second stage of labour after a failed attempt at OVB can be extremely challenging with impaction of the fetal head, extension of the uterine incision and massive obstetric haemorrhage.

Conclusion

Operative vaginal births have an important role to play in modern obstetric care. Women who have an OVB are far more likely to have a spontaneous vaginal birth in a subsequent pregnancy than women who have an emergency caesarean section. Careful patient assessment, observing the rules of safe obstetric practice and working within the appropriate clinical indications for OVBs should ensure that the benefits of recommending OVB outweigh the risks.

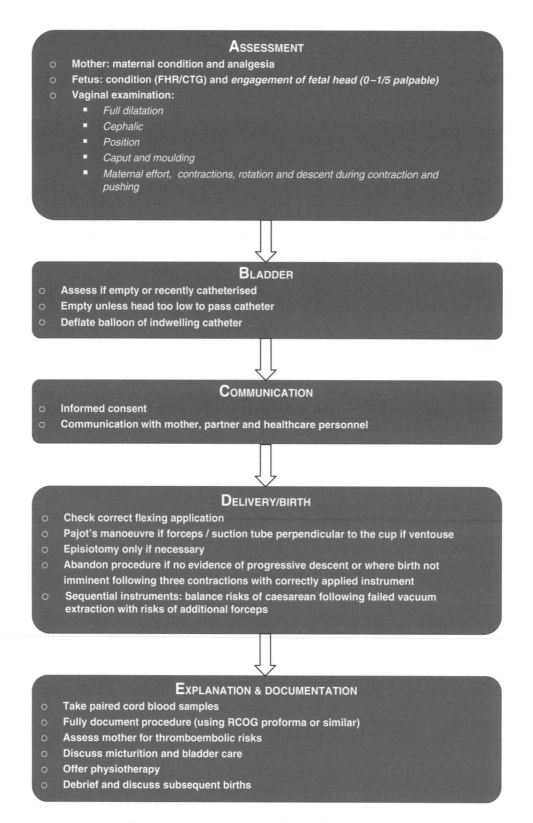

ASSESSMENT
- Mother: maternal condition and analgesia
- Fetus: condition (FHR/CTG) and *engagement of fetal head (0–1/5 palpable)*
- Vaginal examination:
  - *Full dilatation*
  - *Cephalic*
  - *Position*
  - *Caput and moulding*
  - *Maternal effort, contractions, rotation and descent during contraction and pushing*

BLADDER
- Assess if empty or recently catheterised
- Empty unless head too low to pass catheter
- Deflate balloon of indwelling catheter

COMMUNICATION
- Informed consent
- Communication with mother, partner and healthcare personnel

DELIVERY/BIRTH
- Check correct flexing application
- Pajot's manoeuvre if forceps / suction tube perpendicular to the cup if ventouse
- Episiotomy only if necessary
- Abandon procedure if no evidence of progressive descent or where birth not imminent following three contractions with correctly applied instrument
- Sequential instruments: balance risks of caesarean following failed vacuum extraction with risks of additional forceps

EXPLANATION & DOCUMENTATION
- Take paired cord blood samples
- Fully document procedure (using RCOG proforma or similar)
- Assess mother for thromboembolic risks
- Discuss micturition and bladder care
- Offer physiotherapy
- Debrief and discuss subsequent births

Flowchart 2.1 ROBuST flow chart – ABCDE

References

1. Demissie K, Rhoads GG, Smulian JC, Balasubramanian BA, Gandhi K, Joseph KS, et al. Operative vaginal delivery and neonatal and infant adverse outcomes: population based retrospective analysis. *BMJ* 2004;329:24–9.

2. Murphy D, Liebling R, Verity L, Swingler R, Patel R. Cohort study of the early maternal and neonatal morbidity associated with operative delivery in the second stage of labour. *Lancet* 2001; 358:1203–7.

3. DiMatteo MR, Morton SC, Lepper HS, Damush TM, Carney MF, Pearson M, et al. Cesarean childbirth and psychosocial outcomes: a meta-analysis. *Health Psychol* 1996;15:303–14.

4. Bahl R, Strachan B, Murphy DJ. Outcome of subsequent pregnancy three years after previous operative delivery in the second stage of labour: cohort study. *BMJ* 2004;328:311.

5. Cunningham F, Leveno K, Bloom S, Hauth JC, Rouse S, Spong C. *Williams Obstetrics (23rd edition)*. New York: McGraw Hill; 2009. p. 1385.

6. Royal College of Obstetricians and Gynaecologists. *Operative vaginal delivery. Green-top Guideline No. 26*. London: RCOG; 2011.

7. American College of Obstetricians and Gynecologists. *Operative vaginal delivery. ACOG Practice Bulletin 17*. Washington DC: ACOG; 2000.

8. National Institute for Health and Clinical Excellence. *Intrapartum care. Clinical guideline 55*. London: NICE; 2007.

9. Murphy D, Liebling RE, Patel R, Verity L, Swingler R. Cohort study of operative delivery in the second stage of labour and standard of obstetric care. *BJOG*, 2003;110:610–5.

10. Akmal S, Tsoi E, Kametas N, Howard R, Nicolaides KH. Intrapartum sonography to determine fetal head position. *J Matern Fetal Neonatal Med* 2002;12:172–7.

11. Dupuis O, Ruimark S, Corinne D, Simone T, Andre D, Rene-Charles R. Fetal head position during the second stage of labor: Comparison of digital vaginal examination and transabdominal ultrasonographic examination. *Eur J Obstet Gynecol Reprod Biol* 2005;123:193–7.

12. Souka AP, Haritos T, Basayiannis K, Noikokyri N, Antsaklis A. Intrapartum ultrasound for the examination of the fetal head position in normal and obstructed labor. *J Matern Fetal Neonatal Med* 2003;13:59–63.

13. Sherer DM, Miodovnik M, Bradley KS, Langer O. Intrapartum fetal head position II: Comparison between transvaginal digital examination and transabdominal ultrasound assessment during the second stage of labor. *Ultrasound Obstet Gynecol* 2002;19:264–8.

14. Kreiser D, Schiff E, Lipitz S, Kayam A, Avraham A, Achiron R. Determination of fetal occiput position by ultrasound during the second stage of labor. *J Matern Fetal Neonatal Med* 2001;10:283–6.

15. Zahalka N, Sadan O, Malinger G, Liberati M, Boaz M, Glezerman M, et al. Comparison of transvaginal sonography with digital examination and transabdominal sonography for the determination of fetal head position in the second stage of labor. *Am J Obstet Gynecol*, 2005;193:381–6.

16. Chou R, Kreiser D, Taslimi M, Druzin M, El-Sayed Y. Vaginal versus ultrasound examination of fetal occiput position during the second stage of labor. *Am J Obstet Gynecol* 2004;191:521–4.

17. Rozenberg P, Porcher R, Salomon LJ, Boirot F, Morin C, Ville Y. Comparison of the learning curves of digital examination and transabdominal sonography for the determination of fetal head position during labor. *Ultrasound Obstet Gynecol* 2008;31:332–7.

18. Ramphul M, Murphy DJ. Establishing the accuracy and acceptability of abdominal ultrasound to define the fetal head position in the second stage of labour: a validation study. *Eur J Obstet Gynecol Reprod Biol* 2012;164:35–9.

19. Akmal S, Kametas N, Tsoi E, Hargreaves C, Nicolaides KH. Comparison of transvaginal digital examination with intrapartum sonography to determine fetal head position before instrumental delivery. *Ultrasound Obstet Gynecol* 2003;21:437–40.

20. Wong GY, Mok YM, Wong SF. Transabdominal ultrasound assessment of the fetal head and the accuracy of vacuum cup application. *Int J Gynaecol Obstet* 2007;98:120–3.

21. Dupuis O, Silveira R, Zentner A, Dittmar A, Gaucherand P, Cucherat M, et al. Birth simulator: Reliability of transvaginal assessment of fetal head station as defined by the American College of Obstetricians and Gynecologists classification. *Am J Obstet Gynecol* 2005;192:868–74.

22. Barbera AF, Pombar X, Perugino D, Lezotte DC, Hobbins J. A new method to assess fetal head descent in labor with transperineal ultrasound, *Ultrasound Obstet Gynecol*, 2009; 33:313–19.

23. Dietz HP, Lanzarone V, Measuring engagement of the fetal head: validity and reproducibility of a new ultrasound technique. *Ultrasound Obstet Gynecol* 2005;25:165–8.

24. Tutschek B, Braun T, Chantraine F, Henrich W. A study of progress of labour using intrapartum translabial ultrasound, assessing head station, direction, and angle of descent. *BJOG* 2011;118:62–9.

25. Henrich W, Dudenhausen J, Fuchs I, Kamena A, Tutschek B. Intrapartum translabial ultrasound (ITU): sonographic landmarks and correlation with successful vacuum extraction. *Ultrasound Obstet Gynecol* 2006;28:753–60.

26. Awan N, Rhoades A, Weeks AD. The validity and reliability of the StationMaster: a device to improve the accuracy of station assessment in labour. *Eur J Obstet Gynecol Reprod Biol* 2009;145:65–70.

27. O'Mahony F, Hofmeyr GJ, Menon V, Choice of instruments for assisted vaginal delivery. *Cochrane Database Syst Rev*, 2010;(11):CD005455.

28. Patel RR, Murphy DJ. Forceps delivery in modern obstetric practice. *BMJ* 2004;328:1302–5.

29. Murphy D, Macleod M, Bahl R, Strachan B. A cohort study of maternal and neonatal morbidity in relation to use of sequential instruments at operative vaginal delivery. *Eur J Obstet Gynecol Reprod Biol* 2011;156:41–5.

30. Okunwobi-Smith Y, Cooke I, MacKenzie IZ. Decision to delivery intervals for assisted vaginal vertex delivery. *BJOG* 2000;107:467–71.

31. Groom KM, Jones BA, Miller N, Paterson-Brown S. A prospective randomised controlled trial of the Kiwi Omnicup versus conventional ventouse cups for vacuum-assisted vaginal delivery. *BJOG* 2006;113:183–9.

32. Attilakos G, Sibanda T, Winter C, Johnson N, Draycott T. A randomised controlled trial of a new handheld vacuum extraction device. *BJOG* 2005;112:1510–15.

33. Murphy DJ, Koh DK. Cohort study of the decision to delivery interval and neonatal outcome for emergency operative vaginal delivery. *Am J Obstet Gynecol* 2007;196:145, e1–7.

34. Spencer C, Murphy D, Bewley S. Caesarean delivery in the second stage of labour. *BMJ* 2006;333:613–4.

Chapter 3
Nontechnical skills

Bryony Strachan and Rachna Bahl

> ## Key learning points
>
> - To define and explain the importance of nontechnical skills in obstetric practice.
> - To describe the nontechnical skills useful when conducting operative vaginal birth (OVB).
> - To describe examples of good behaviours.

Well I guess when you think of forceps and ventouse ... it just sounds very scary and having your feet up in stirrups and just lying there not feeling anything ... having lots of people whizzing all around you, it is quite scary you sort of feel like "a piece of meat on a butcher's table" in a way you do feel quite helpless because you just have to ... you're at the mercy of the doctors having to hope they're doing their best in a way.

A mother.

The components of a good OVB are complex and layered. They go far beyond a degree of knowledge and technical ability. They encompass a range of cognitive and social skills that promote respect for women and their partners and enable an environment in which women feel safe and are secure, acknowledging her rite of passage and the privilege of assisting at the birth of a new life. This chapter explores our understanding of these important 'nontechnical' skills of a consummate accoucheur.

What are nontechnical skills?

Nontechnical skills are cognitive and social skills required in an operational task involving decision making and team work.[1] These are distinct skills, separate from an obstetrician's knowledge of the instruments and the technique and manual dexterity. These skills or lack of them have been identified as contributors to a significant proportion of adverse events in health care.[2,3] A study of adverse events in surgery identified communication as the causal factor in 43% of errors made.[4] Similar findings have been identified in obstetrics. A joint commission into the study of errors in obstetric care concluded that failure of team work and communication were the cause of 70% of adverse events.[5] The effect of decision making has been studied extensively and has been shown to have a direct effect on safety.[6–8]

Nontechnical skills have been studied in surgical, anaesthetic and acute medicine domains using methodology from the aviation industry.[9–12] Operative vaginal birth (OVB) merits nontechnical skills unique to this very intimate and emotive time for the mother and her birth partner. Unlike the scenarios studied in anaesthesia and surgery, the mother is awake and her cooperation and confidence in the caregivers can influence the outcome of the procedure. In the vast majority of cases, the decision to conduct an OVB is made in the second stage of labour when the mother is arguably at her most vulnerable. Operative vaginal birth is considered a deviation from natural childbirth which the mother generally believes to be the utopian or ideal way of giving birth.[13] Operative birth, dissatisfaction with antenatal care and the presence of unwanted personnel in the labour room have all been associated with a greater risk of postnatal depression among mothers.[14] Therefore, the obstetrician needs to be aware of not only the cognitive but also the social and interactive nontechnical skills required when performing an OVB.

Classification of nontechnical skills

A three-tier behavioural system is used to classify nontechnical skills. The first level has five major categories of these skills.[9–11] When conducting an OVB, the main categories to be considered are:

- situational awareness
- decision making
- team work and communication
- professional relationships with the woman
- maintaining professional behaviour.

Table 3.1 Nontechnical skills required for operative vaginal birth

Category	Element
Cognitive skills	
Situational awareness	Gather information
	Understand and analyse information
	Anticipate hazards
	Plan contingencies
Decision making	Consider all options
	Implement one option
	Evaluate/reassess the option chosen
Social skills	
Team work and communication	Clear exchange of information
	Identify resources
	Be aware of team capabilities
	Have respect for members of the team
	Cross-check: be a 'wing man'
Professional relationship with the woman	Communicate with the mother
	Maintain respect for and ensure dignity of the mother
	Partner participation
Maintaining professional behaviour	Calm
	Confident/assertive
	Able

Each category is subdivided into elements. The elements define observable individual skills. For each element identified examples of good behaviour are described.

Table 3.1 describes skills for an individual obstetrician rather than the multidisciplinary team. The reason for defining the skills for an individual is to enable each team member to be aware of his/her training needs in their domain. If all team members have good nontechnical skills relevant to their area of expertise, the team is likely to function efficiently. Moreover, healthcare practitioners work in temporary teams and the team members change with every shift. Therefore, individual skills need to be addressed as well as the team nontechnical skills.

When describing nontechnical skills for training, they are divided into two main groups.

- **Cognitive skills** such as situational awareness and decision making. Good problem solving, sound judgement and effective decision making are considered among the highest attributes of clinicians.[15]

- **Social skills** such as team working, communication, maintaining a professional behaviour and developing a professional relationship with the mother. These skills are not new to obstetricians, and experienced obstetricians have always demonstrated these skills as an integral part of their practice. However, it is important that trainee obstetricians are aware of these observable skills because they can have a significant impact on the physical and psychological outcomes of the OVB.

Categories of nontechnical skills

Situational awareness

Situational awareness is defined as the perception of elements in the environment, comprehension of their meaning and the projection of their status in the near future.[16] It essentially means that the operator is aware of what is going on and how it can affect the outcome. The term situational awareness was first used in military and has since been used in the aviation industry. It was introduced to medicine in anaesthetics when crew resource management training used in aviation was used as a model for team training in anaesthesia.[17] A good pilot will be 'ahead of the plane' and have planned his/her route, acknowledging potential hazards such as weather patterns or an unusual airport approach or mechanical factors for which he/she has planned contingencies so the flight is smooth and uneventful. Likewise, a good obstetrician will be 'ahead of the labour ward' and will have an up-to-date briefing of the labour ward board, anticipating which women may need obstetric help and when, will have an understanding of staffing matters and will have planned for contingencies. Situational awareness is an important skill in conducting a safe instrumental birth. Gathering appropriate information and assimilating it to make the decision that provides the best option for mother and baby is vital in minimising the morbidity associated with OVB. Situational awareness enables the obstetrician to make an appropriate decision when deciding whether an OVB is indicated and, if indicated, where it should be conducted and what should be the instrument of choice.

Examples of good practice: situational awareness

Information gathering:

- reviews the antenatal history and progress in labour
- reviews maternal and fetal wellbeing
- conducts abdominal and vaginal examination
- cross-checks information and checks the state of the labour ward.

Understanding and analysing information:

- identifies risk factors predisposing to a need for OVB
- identifies factors that can help reduce the likelihood of OVB.

Anticipation:

- implements factors to facilitate normal birth where applicable
- anticipates complexity of the planned OVB and takes relevant actions
- anticipates potential complications and has planned contingencies, e.g. for increased risk of failure to deliver or postpartum haemorrhage.

Various situational awareness strategies have been shown to reduce the likelihood of requiring an OVB in order to promote a spontaneous birth. Continuous support during labour, use of upright or lateral positions, avoiding epidural and delayed pushing in primiparous women with an epidural can reduce the need for an OVB. When called to review a mother with a view to conducting an OVB, in the absence of suspected fetal distress, certain strategies can be considered to avoid an OVB (Figure 3.1).

Decision making

Decision making is the process of reaching a judgement or choosing an option to meet the needs of a given situation.[15] It is a cyclical process where an action is selected and continually re-evaluated. Any deviation from anticipated progression leads to change in action to achieve the optimum result.

The behavioural markers for the three elements of decision-making skill are shown below. The trainees should become familiar with these behavioural markers when training in simulation or when dealing with nonurgent clinical situations. Familiarity with the decision-making elements will enable the obstetricians to implement these processes in stressful clinical situations and facilitate them to make appropriate decisions.

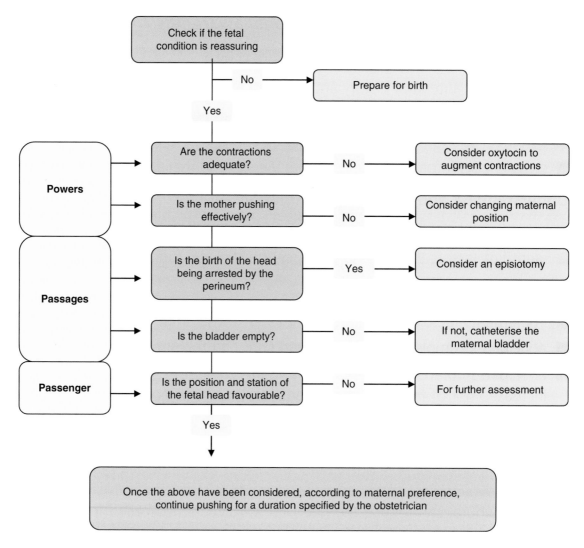

Figure 3.1 Strategies to improve spontaneous birth

Examples of good practice: decision making

Consider all available options:

- generates the options of whether to conduct the birth in the labour room or in the operating theatre in the context of the clinical situation
- generates the options of various instruments that can be used to conduct the birth
- discusses the options with the mother and her partner.

Implement one option:

- considers the risks and benefits of various options and selects the most appropriate option
- implements the selected option with in the timescale selected.

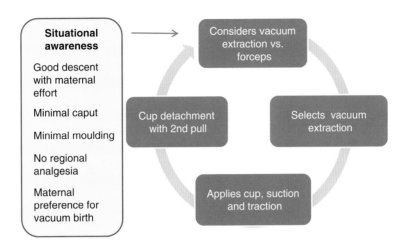

Figure 3.2 Decision making for selecting an appropriate instrument for OVB

Evaluate/reassess the option chosen:

■ reviews the progress at each step
■ if progress not as anticipated, takes further actions such as:
    ☐ call for senior support
    ☐ change the course of OVB
    ☐ abandon procedure.

An example of use of the above elements of decision making when selecting an appropriate instrument for OVB is shown in Figure 3.2. The obstetrician needs to consider the cues from situational awareness when making a decision about the most appropriate instrument for conducting the OVB. Once the instrument has been selected and the procedure has begun, it is important to reassess at each step. In the scenario detailed above, there were no deviations from the anticipated progress until the traction was applied for the second time. At this stage the cup detached from the fetal scalp. This situation prompts the obstetrician to reassess the clinical situation. The decision regarding further action will be based on the most likely cause for cup detachment and the likelihood of achieving a vaginal birth.

Team work and communication

The most commonly known nontechnical skills are team work and communication. Team working is the skill of working in a group of health professionals and ensuring that the efforts are directed at reaching the common goal. As a team worker the focus is not only on the task but also on the team members.

Exchange of information is vital when coordinating the team to perform a task. This helps in gathering information (situational awareness) and selecting the most appropriate action (decision making). Communication can be verbal or nonverbal, but it is important that the message being communicated is explicit and unambiguous. The purpose of the communication is that the message is received and understood by the team member it is directed at. Poor communication not only compromises team morale and safety, it is also noticeable to the mother. It has been reported that poor communication between the health professionals can lead to dissatisfaction with the care a mother receives during childbirth.[19] Once the decision for conducting an OVB is made, the obstetrician should communicate clearly to the midwife looking after the mother and the midwife in charge of the labour ward.

One should be aware not only of one's own ability but also the capability of the team. Obstetricians are often aware of or make an effort to establish the ability of a trainee they are supervising. However, it is also important to ensure that the midwife is aware of her/his role in this scenario and her role has been communicated to her/him clearly. If the midwife needs support, this should be identified and arranged. A good team is one in which the members support each other. If one is not aware of the limitations of the team members, it can often become difficult to limit harm done by the less able professional. All of us will need a support and a 'wing man' to look out for us at some time. One of the cornerstones of team working is that team members have mutual respect for each other. This holds true for the team working when conducting an OVB. It is important for team morale and performance that the team members are treated in a manner that makes them feel respected and valued. If a conflict arises, every effort should be made to resolve it instantly. Below are the behavioural markers identified for obstetricians in the context of OVB.

Examples of good practice: team work and communication

Clear exchange of information:

- informs the midwife caring for the woman of the urgency, instrument and the place of birth
- discusses with the midwife in charge of the labour ward and ensures that OVB is appropriately prioritised in relation to the workload on the labour ward.

Identify resources:

- ensures all the necessary equipment is available
- ensures that the instruments are available easily on the trolley
- ensures that all the personnel are present and ready for the birth
- delegates tasks clearly.

Aware of team capabilities:

- ensures that the midwife in the room understands her/his role
- ensures that the midwife is competent and confident about her/his role in the birth.

Respect for team members:

- is polite to the team members when asking for equipment
- registers and acknowledges their opinion
- debriefs and thanks team after a difficult birth.

Professional relationship with the woman and her birthing partner

This category does not feature in the taxonomy of surgical nontechnical skills and is unique to obstetrics. During labour and birth the woman and her partner are aware of the proceedings in the room and anticipate full participation. In the study into nontechnical skills of obstetricians conducting OVB, this category was considered extremely important by obstetricians and midwives. The elements that form this category arguably constitute the behaviours a woman is likely to remember and these behaviours will have a great impact on her perception of the birth. Communication with the mother is the main building block for developing a professional relationship with her.

Examples of good practice: professional relationship with the woman

Communication with the mother:

- introduces him/herself to the mother and her partner
- explains what his/her role is and why asked to review
- explains the proposed procedure clearly and in easy to understand terms

- explains the commonly anticipated complications
- listens to the mother's concerns and attempts to address them
- tailors care to the mother's wishes, such as preference for a particular instrument
- obtains informed consent.

Maintain the dignity of the mother:

- makes an effort to cover the mother
- keeps the door to the delivery room closed
- minimises unnecessary visits to the room
- asks and uses the mother's preferred name.

Partner participation:

- involves the birthing partner in the decision-making process.

Maintaining professional behaviour

This category is considered a vital nontechnical skill by obstetricians and midwives. The elements discussed here are described as key leadership skills when detailing nontechnical skills in other domains. A team leader is defined as a person who is appointed, elected or informally chosen to direct or coordinate the work of others in a group.[18] However, during the study of nontechnical skills of obstetricians conducting an OVB, it was felt that the above definition did not always apply to the obstetrician. The leader of the procedure of the OVB is sometimes not the leader of the complete clinical situation. This becomes apparent when a junior trainee is conducting the OVB and a senior midwife is maintaining situational awareness and leadership of the whole clinical scenario. The clinical situation where the patient is actively involved throughout the procedure brings another dimension to this category. The boundary between assertiveness and aggressiveness is sometimes blurred when leading a task. However, with OVB, it is essential that the obstetrician is assertive but not aggressive towards the team or the mother. Therefore, the category is named 'maintaining professional behaviour'.

One of the common indications for OVB is suspected fetal compromise. This is an anxious time for the mother and it is therefore essential that the obstetrician appears calm and in control. As the obstetrician is leading the team, his/her attitude will have an influence on how everyone else in the room perceives the situation. A junior trainee may not be confident about performing the procedure. The trainee should be aware of his/her limitations, but it is important that the lack of confidence is not apparent when conducting the birth. It is also important that the obstetrician appears able and assertive during the birth.

Examples of good practice: maintaining professional behaviour

Calm:

- stays calm in an emergency situation
- does not appear stressed.

Confident/assertive:

- creates a confident atmosphere
- provides clear, firm instructions
- takes the lead.

Able:

- knows his/her limitations
- is open and honest about his/her ability and reflects on the experience
- is gentle and shows empathy.

Discussion

Operative vaginal birth requires complex technical and nontechnical skills. The decision-making processes become more challenging when the information is incomplete and the clinical situation highly emotive.[19,20] Decision aids can be used to reduce the relative effort needed for making a decision. Knowledge of the principles of situational awareness and explicit decision-making skills can aid trainees' understanding of when to intervene, where best to conduct the birth and the optimal choice of instrument for an OVB in relation to clinical assessment in the second stage of labour.

The social and interpersonal skills not only contribute to patient safety but also can lead to a lasting impression on the mother. Therefore, the value of these should not be underestimated and need to be carefully built into teaching and formative assessments.

Classification of skills into categories and elements is helpful when developing a training package as well as to structure feedback to trainee obstetricians. Use of simulation and video feedback can be useful to discuss these skills with trainees.

The limitation of this behavioural marker system is that it describes individual skills that are easy to observe and does not include every cognitive skill. We have focused on the observable skills because the main aim is to use the system for future training.

References

1. Fletcher GC, McGeorge P, Flin RH, Glavin RJ, Maran NJ. The role of non-technical skills in anaesthesia: a review of current literature. *Br J Anaesth* 2002;88:418–29.

2. Bogner M (editor). *Human error in medicine*. Hillsdale, NJ: LEA; 1994.

3. Bogner M (editor). *Misadventures in health care*. Mahwah, NJ: LEA; 2004.

4. Wilson J. *A practical guide to risk management in surgery; developing and planning*. Healthcare Risk Resources International – Royal College of Surgeons Symposium 1999.

5. Guise JM, Segel S. Teamwork in obstetric critical care. *Best Pract Res Clin Obstet Gynaecol* 2008;22:937–51.

6. Helmriech RL, Foushee HC. Why crew resource management? Empirical and theoretical bases of human factor training in aviation. In: Weiner EL, Kanki BG, Helmriech RL (editors). *Cockpit Resource Management*. London: Academic Press; 1993. pp. 3–45.

7. Flin R, Salas E, Strub M, Martin L. *Decision making under stress*. Aldershot: Ashgate; 1997.

8. Montgomery H, Lipshitz R, Brehmer B. *How professionals make decisions*. Mahwah, NJ: Lawrence Erlbaum; 2005.

9. Flin R, Maran N. Identifying and training non-technical skills for teams in acute medicine. *Qual Saf Health Care*. 2004;13 Suppl 1:i80–4.

10. Fletcher G, Flin R, McGeorge P, Glavin R, Maran N, Patey R. Anaesthetists' Non-Technical Skills (ANTS): evaluation of a behavioural marker system. *Br J Anaesth* 2003;90:580–8.

11. Yule S, Flin R, Paterson-Brown S, Maran N, Rowley D. Development of a rating system for surgeons' non-technical skills. *Med Educ* 2006;40:1098–104.

12. McCulloch P, Mishra A, Handa A, Dale T, Hirst G, Catchpole K. The effects of aviation-style non-technical skills training on technical performance and outcome in the operating theatre. *Qual Saf Health Care* 2009;18:109–15.

13. Frost J. Pope C, Liebling R, Murphy D. Utopian theory and the discourse of natural birth. *Social Theory & Health* 2006;4:299–318.

14. Astbury J, Brown S, Lumley J, Small R. Birth events, birth experiences and social differences in postnatal depression. *Aust J Public Health* 1994;18:176–84.

15. Croskerry P. The theory and practice of clinical decision-making. *Can J Anaesth* 2005;52:R1–8.

16. Endsley M. Towards a theory of situational awareness in dynamic systems. *Human Factors* 1995;37:32–64.

17. Gaba D, Howard S, Small S. Situational awareness in anesthesiology. *Human Factors*. 1995;37:20–31.

18. TNS for the COI Communications (on behalf of Department of Health). *NHS Maternity Services Quantitative Research*, The Stationery Office, October 2005. Available at: www.dh.gov. uk/assetRoot;?04/12/42/44/04/12422.pdf (accessed July 2012).

19. Bowen J. Educational strategies to promote clinical diagonostic reasoning. *N Engl J Med* 2006;355:2217–25.

20. Charlin B, Boshuizen HP, Custers EJ, Feltovich PJ. Scripts and clinical reasoning. *Med Educ* 2007;41:1178–84.

Chapter 4
Vacuum-assisted birth

Aldo Vacca

Key learning points

■ Importance of the flexion point in vacuum-assisted birth and how to achieve correct cup application to the fetal head.

■ Technique to reduce failure and cup detachment rates with attempted vacuum-assisted birth.

■ Technical aspects to improve the safety of vacuum-assisted birth for the mother and newborn infant.

When a valid indication for vacuum-assisted birth exists, the relevant obstetric variables should be identified and carefully assessed to determine whether vacuum-assisted birth is appropriate and safe under the clinical circumstances and for the level of experience of the operator. This important decision-making process is considered in other chapters of the book. This chapter focuses on a few selected technical matters that should, if followed, improve the efficacy and reduce the risk of vacuum-assisted birth.

Essential principles for vacuum-assisted birth

The flexion point and midpoint of the fetal head

The flexion point is an imaginary point on the sagittal suture of the fetal scalp, 3 cm anterior to (i.e. in front of) the posterior fontanelle.[1] It marks the exit point of the mentovertical diameter and is a critical landmark for vacuum-assisted birth. When the centre of a vacuum cup has been placed over

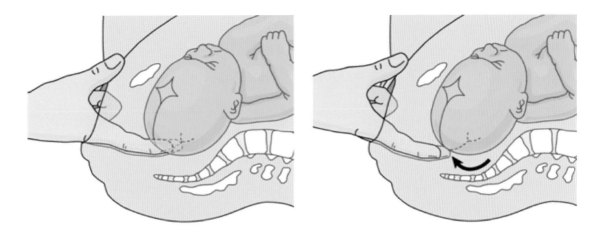

Figure 4.1 Locating the flexion point

the flexion point and axis traction is applied, fetal head diameters will be optimal for birth. Regardless of the position of the head, the operator should be able to locate the flexion point and correctly position the cup over it (Figure 4.1).

The midpoint of the fetal head is situated on the mentovertical diameter but within the cranium approximately 6 cm from the vertex. Its significance lies in the fact that the long axis of the fetal head pivots at the level of the midpoint as the head descends. Therefore, traction with a vacuum extractor should not be directed upwards until the midpoint has passed beneath the symphysis pubis. Furthermore, since the midpoint is situated at the same level as the widest diameters of the fetal head, the resistance to birth is greatest at this level and not at the level of the cup. The implication for practice is that when the vacuum cup has reached the vaginal introitus the widest diameters of the fetal head are passing through the narrowest part of the birth canal, namely the pelvic floor and perineum. This phase of a vacuum-assisted birth is generally associated with higher resistance levels than those encountered during the descent phase.[2]

Choice of suitable vacuum cup

The design of a vacuum cup is the major factor that determines its manoeuvrability within the lower birth canal and therefore its appropriate clinical use.[1] Vacuum cups that are commercially available include:

- Soft 'anterior' cups (plastic or rubber):
  - ☐ Silc and silastic cups
  - ☐ Mystic MitySoft cup
  - ☐ Kiwi ProCup

- Rigid 'anterior' cups (plastic or metal):
  - ☐ Malmström, Bird and O'Neil anterior cups
  - ☐ Kiwi OmniCup (anterior mode)
  - ☐ M-Style Mystic Mityvac cup
- Rigid 'posterior' cups (plastic or metal):
  - ☐ Bird and O'Neil posterior cups
  - ☐ Kiwi OmniCup (posterior mode)
  - ☐ M-Select Mityvac cup

The rigid anterior cups (metal and plastic) and all soft cups are suitable if the occiput is anterior and the fetal station is low or at the outlet. A posterior cup should be used for all occipito-transverse (OT) and occipito-posterior (OP) positions and for oblique anterior positions when the scalp is not visible between contractions.

The five steps of a vacuum-assisted birth

1. Locating the flexion point and calculating the cup-insertion distance

Before applying the cup to the fetal head, the position of the occiput is rechecked and the precise location of the flexion point is confirmed.[3] The cup insertion distance can then be estimated by using the middle finger of the examining hand (Figure 4.2). This calculation should be made during the vaginal examination conducted as part of the assessment of labour.

2. Holding and inserting the cup

The operator lightly smears the outside of the vacuum cup with obstetric cream and gently retracts the perineum with two fingers to form a space into which the cup is inserted with one movement immediately following a contraction. Posterior cups should be held with the thumb on the dome of the cup and two fingers on the rim nearest the operator. The rigid anterior cups are held in the hand near the suction tube's attachment to the cup and the soft cups are grasped near the broad flexible end and compressed to make insertion easier.

3. Manoeuvring the cup toward the flexion point

For low and outlet occipito-anterior (OA) positions, the flexion point will be located in or near the introitus and little manoeuvring of the cup will be necessary to achieve a flexing median application. At low and outlet stations,

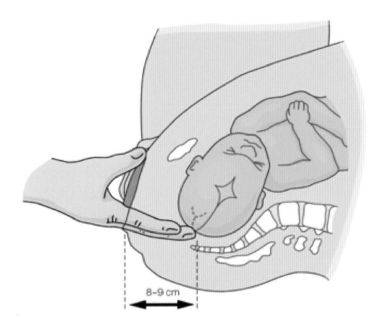

8–9 cm

Figure 4.2 Low OT, with asynclitism; digital distance 8–9 cm

the vagina sweeps around the lower part of the fetal head and the labia minora may fall across the vaginal introitus. As a result, these tissues may be at risk of entrapment beneath the vacuum cup. To avoid this problem, one hand holds the cup in position against the fetal head while the index finger of the other hand is swept around the periphery of the cup to exclude maternal tissue.

For mid- and low-pelvic OP and OT positions, the flexion point will be displaced away from the introitus towards the sacrum and considerable manoeuvring of the cup will be required to achieve a correct application. Therefore, a manoeuvrable posterior-design cup should be selected for vacuum-assisted births where the fetal head is malpositioned. Displacement of the flexion point in OP and OT positions is mainly in an anteroposterior direction of the birth canal and, to a lesser extent, laterally. For practical purposes, therefore, the posterior cup should be manoeuvred in the mother's midline pelvic axis to the flexion point.[3]

In OP and OT positions of the head it is usually not possible to reach the distal part of a correctly placed cup to exclude maternal tissue entrapment. In these cases the vagina is being pushed outwards by the widest diameters of the fetal head and insertion of the cup into the space between the head and pelvic floor will distend the vagina even further. For this reason, maternal entrapment under the cup is unlikely. Operators should therefore check for tissue entrapment along the reachable margins of the cup nearest the introitus. Too vigorous an attempt to reach the distal parts of the cup may cause maternal discomfort or may dislodge the cup.

4. Inducing and maintaining the vacuum

When the operator is satisfied that the cup has been applied over the flexion point, the recommended vacuum pressure of 60–80 kPa may be attained in one step.[4] However, if the operator is not confident that the cup has been placed correctly, it is advisable to pause when a vacuum of 20 kPa has been reached to check the application and to exclude vaginal tissue entrapment.

Gentle traction may be started as soon as a contraction begins and the mother begins to push, but stronger traction should be delayed for 1 minute to allow the chignon to completely form. Some operators reduce the vacuum to a lower level between contractions, although the evidence has not demonstrated any benefits for the fetus from this technique,[5] nor is there any evidence to support the view that levels of negative pressure below 80 kPa are associated with a reduction in scalp injury. For these reasons, it would seem preferable to maintain the vacuum at working levels until the head has been delivered.

5. Method of traction

The operator should kneel on one knee or sit on a low stool so that traction can be applied in a downward direction along the axis of the pelvis. For low extractions when the scalp becomes visible or when the head has descended to the outlet, the direction of traction will change progressively in an upwards direction until the standing position becomes more appropriate.

Traction should be performed as a two-handed exercise with both hands working in unison: one providing the traction (the 'pulling' hand) and the other monitoring the progress and providing countertraction when necessary (the 'nonpulling' hand) (Figure 4.3). Traction with the vacuum extractor should be regarded as an adjunct to the expulsive forces of labour and not as the primary means of overcoming resistance to descent. If contractions are weak or infrequent, oxytocin infusion should be instituted promptly because the number, duration and strength of pulls required for birth are inversely proportional to the efficiency of the contractions and maternal effort.

The 'finger-tip' position of the pulling hand

Vacuum devices that are fitted with or incorporate a traction bar or handle should be held with the bar cradled in the slightly flexed distal interphalangeal joints with the palm of the hand opened and facing upwards (Figure 4.3). In most cases sufficient traction for birth of the infant can be generated

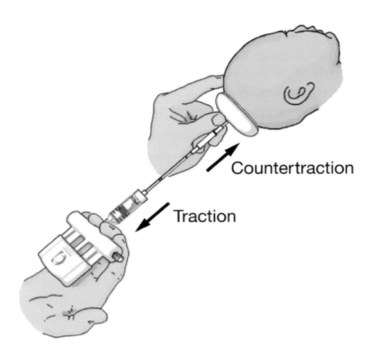

Figure 4.3 The two-handed traction technique

simply by flexing the fingers that are holding the bar. The principal functions of the pulling hand are to direct traction along the axis of the pelvis so that fetal presenting diameters are optimal for birth, i.e. axis traction; to provide additional but not excessive traction to complement the mother's expulsive powers; to limit the traction force by pulling with the finger tips; and to pull only when the uterus is contracting and the mother is pushing.

The 'finger–thumb' position of the nonpulling hand

The standard position for the nonpulling hand should be with the thumb placed on the dome of the cup, providing some degree of counterpressure when required during traction, and with the index finger of the same hand resting on the fetal scalp in front of the cup to monitor progress at the level of the midpoint of the head. Since most cup detachments occur when the cup is visible at the vaginal introitus, the finger–thumb position must be maintained until the head has crowned or delivered to reduce the risk of detachment. Therefore, if perineal support (guarding) is practised, this should be provided by an assistant and not by the operator.

The principal functions of the nonpulling hand are to monitor progress with each pull – descent, flexion and autorotation – of the fetal head; to control the traction force transmitted to the fetal scalp by varying the amount of counterpressure with the thumb; to avoid complete detachment ('pop off') of the cup by counterpressure with the thumb; and to serve as a rotary point for the completion of autorotation by slowing progress across the perineum.

Axis traction with the vacuum extractor should result in progressive descent of the head with the least amount of traction force. Attachment of the cup to the scalp has been shown to be most effective when the direction of pull is perpendicular to the cup.[6] This is almost always possible during vacuum-assisted birth except in the initial stages in OP and OT positions when the head is deflexed or asynclitic. However, gentle downward traction will quickly correct the attitude of the head, after which perpendicular traction can be achieved. Oblique traction is a factor associated with difficult vacuum-assisted birth and cup detachment, which predispose to scalp injury. Rocking movements from side to side[7] or manually turning the rigid handles of some cups[8] is not recommended because the shearing force or torque associated with such practices may increase the predisposition for cup detachment and fetal scalp injury.

Traction should commence at the onset of a contraction with the mother bearing down and should be maintained as long as she is pushing. The operator should offer encouragement to the mother and inform her of the progress she is making. Some mothers prefer to push in two or three shorter episodes during the contraction. In these circumstances, the operator should cease pulling when the mother stops pushing and recommence traction when she resumes expulsive efforts. As soon as the contraction passes or the mother stops pushing, traction should be ceased. Traction should not be continued between contractions; traction to 'maintain station' during the interval to prevent retraction of the head should not be applied because the force on the head, without maternal propulsive effort, may injure the fetal scalp or the mother's pelvic floor. Descent achieved at the end of one contraction will quickly be re-gained at the start of the next contraction. During the procedure the fetal heart should be monitored regularly by continuous external electronic monitoring or by an assistant using a hand-held device following each contraction.

The descent phase and the pelvic floor phase of a vacuum-assisted birth

It is advisable to consider vacuum-assisted birth as a two-phase procedure: a descent phase and a pelvic floor/perineal phase.[2] The descent phase is that part of the vacuum extraction from application of the cup until the cup has descended to and is completely visible in the vaginal introitus. This marks the start of the pelvic floor phase, which lasts until completion of the birth of the fetal head. In a prospective study of vacuum-assisted birth in nulliparous women, higher levels of traction force and a greater number of pulls were recorded in the majority of cases during the pelvic floor and perineal phase than during the descent phase.[2] The explanation may be that during the pelvic floor phase the widest diameters of the fetal head are negotiating the narrowest part of the maternal birth canal.

Signs of progress

Operators should expect some progress to occur with each pull. Signs of progress are descent of the presenting part, flexion and correction of asynclitism and autorotation of the head in malpositions. When the head is deflexed or asynclitic, the first observed sign is usually flexion and descent of the head. This is evidenced by a visible increase in length of the tube or traction cord outside the vagina. Autorotation will be observed to some degree at all levels as the head descends. The head, not just the scalp, must begin to move with the first pull and some descent should occur with each subsequent pull. Tractions that do not cause the head to descend ('negative' tractions[9]) must be differentiated from those that do, as they are more likely to cause subgaleal haemorrhage. Placing a limit on the number of pulls has been a principal safety measure recommended for avoiding injury to the newborn infant. For this reason, the concept of the 'three pulls rule' was introduced.[10] The rule states 'If there is not good progress after the third pull, the case should be carefully reassessed'. When the rule was proposed, there were no epidurals, mothers were not pushing for long periods in the second stage and episiotomies were performed more liberally. Changes that have occurred in these obstetric practices over more recent times have important implications for vacuum-assisted birth. For this reason, the author recommends allowing three pulls for the descent phase and three pulls for the pelvic floor and perineal phase.[1]

After the birth

After birth of the head, the vacuum is released and the birth is completed in the normal manner. Operators should always forewarn the parents prior to removal of the cup about the appearance of the chignon and reassure them that the swelling will resolve quickly and any marking caused by the cup will disappear completely. As soon as possible after the birth the operator should palpate the area over the chignon with the fingertips to exclude possible subgaleal bleeding. This is particularly important if the birth was difficult or associated with cup detachment. A fluid 'thrill' will sometimes be palpable under the cup application site if the scalp has been separated from the underlying cranium. This small collection is derived from the fluid of the natural caput and chignon, which enters the subgaleal space. Continued bleeding from damaged blood vessels may subsequently result in a subgaleal haematoma. The neonatal paediatric team should be informed of any concerns, especially if difficulty was experienced during the extraction, so that regular inspections of the scalp will be made. In this way, subgaleal bleeding will be detected early, allowing prompt and effective therapy to be instigated.

On the day after the birth, the operator should re-examine the baby in the mother's presence to answer questions she may wish to ask and to allay any concerns she may express about the baby or the birth. In addition, it is an opportune time to discuss the reasons for the procedure and any other aspects that may require consideration in a subsequent pregnancy. If the scalp was injured during the birth, appropriate arrangements should be made for follow-up of the infant. Details of the procedure and the maternal and fetal outcomes should be accurately described in an operative vaginal birth form designed to record relevant data about the procedure and to facilitate regular clinical audit.[11]

Rotational vacuum-assisted birth

Provided the operator has been adequately trained in the use of a posterior cup, the technique of rotational vacuum-assisted birth is identical to the five-step method described for nonrotational vacuum-assisted birth.[3] The complexity of a rotational vacuum procedure arises not from the technique itself but from the clinical circumstances associated with these procedures. Anterior rotation of the malpositioned fetal head during vacuum extraction occurs automatically as a passive event similar to the internal rotation that is part of the mechanism of normal labour. No attempt should be made to manually rotate the head either by manipulating the cup or by grasping a rigid handle and physically rotating the device. An important but little appreciated fact in vacuum-assisted birth is the relationship between correct cup placement and autorotation of the fetal head. It has been demonstrated that autorotation rates of 90% or better can be achieved with vacuum extractions undertaken for OP and OT positions of the head provided the application of the cup causes flexion.[12]

Difficulty, cup detachment and failure to achieve birth

Detachment of the cup may occur for one or more of the following reasons:

- deflexing or paramedian cup applications
- incorrect traction technique, pulling too hard, in the wrong direction or with a rocking motion
- not providing counterpressure on the cup with the thumb during traction
- upwards traction before the midpoint of the head has passed beneath the pubic arch
- not allowing sufficient time for the perineum to stretch over the advancing fetal head, especially if episiotomy is not performed
- a large caput succedaneum or maternal tissue or scalp electrode trapped under the cup
- inadequate vacuum pressure or faulty equipment.

Traction should be discontinued between contractions if an audible 'hiss' is heard signalling loss of vacuum and imminent cup detachment (pop-off). Incorrect application of the cup (deflexing or paramedian), pulling too hard and pulling in the wrong direction are common causes of cup detachment. Cup detachment may injure the scalp and should not be regarded as a safety mechanism of the vacuum extractor.[9] High detachment rates may reflect either problems with the instrument or with the way the instrument is used. The detached cup should be reapplied only if the operator is convinced that the cause of the detachment is not cephalopelvic disproportion and that the scalp has not been injured. If detachment recurs or if the head fails to descend with traction, the procedure should be abandoned and the birth completed by caesarean section if the detachment occurs during the descent phase. However, most cup detachments occur when the cup is visible at or passing through the vaginal introitus. At this stage, the widest diameters of the fetal head, situated some 6 cm or 7 cm behind the cup, are at the level of the mother's resistant pelvic floor and strong traction may result in a cup detachment. Cup detachment may be prevented if the operator controls the rate of progress of the head across the perineum with counterpressure on the cup to give the perineum time to stretch over the advancing head. Upwards traction before the midpoint has passed beneath the symphysis pubis is another common cause of cup detachment. Placing a limit on the number of detachments has been recommended as a safety measure to protect the fetus against serious injury.

Some authorities accept three cup detachments as the upper limit[13] whereas it is the author's recommendation to cease the procedure after two cup detachments.

Studies comparing vacuum extraction and forceps birth have consistently shown that the vacuum extractor is less likely than forceps to complete the birth.[14,15] A number of predisposing factors have been linked to failed vacuum extractions with or without cup detachment. They include OP and OT positions of the head,[16] midcavity procedures,[11] deflexing and paramedian applications of the cup,[12] use of soft cups in preference to rigid cups,[14] extractions attempted before full dilatation of the cervix[11] and cephalopelvic disproportion.[16]

Failure of vacuum extraction with sequential use of forceps to complete the birth has been associated with increased risk of injury to the fetus[17,18] and to the maternal genital tract.[18,19] For these reasons, attempted forceps birth following a failed vacuum extraction is not recommended and should be avoided unless the failure occurs with the head visible at the outlet of the pelvis.[11] However, in four randomised controlled trials in the Cochrane Database of Systematic Reviews[14] and two recent additional UK trials[20,21] with a combined total of 1205 attempted vacuum-assisted births, 264 of the attempts failed (22%). Of the 264 failed vacuum-assisted births, 202 (76%) were subsequently delivered vaginally by forceps without any reported serious injury to the infants or mothers. This suggests that incorrect technique may have been a factor in a number of the births and that most of the failures occurred at the outlet of the pelvis.

Effects on the newborn infant

It is useful for counselling and auditing purposes to classify the effects of vacuum-assisted birth on the newborn infant in terms of their severity and clinical significance. A suggested classification is presented here:

- cosmetic effects:
  - ☐ the chignon (artificial caput succedaneum)
  - ☐ cup discoloration and marking of the scalp
- clinically nonsignificant injuries:
  - ☐ blisters and superficial scalp abrasions
  - ☐ cephalhaematoma
  - ☐ retinal haemorrhage

- clinically significant injuries:
  - ☐ extensive scalp lacerations
  - ☐ subgaleal (subaponeurotic) haemorrhage
  - ☐ intracranial haemorrhage
  - ☐ skull fracture
- indirect and coincidental injuries:
  - ☐ brachial plexus injury
  - ☐ fracture of the clavicle or humerus.

Examination of the data in the current Cochrane Systematic Review[14] demonstrates that soft cups caused fewer cosmetic effects, scalp lacerations and cephalhaematomas than rigid cups. However, all of these effects are transient and do not pose threats to the wellbeing of the infant. There is no evidence to show that soft cups are associated with a reduction in clinically significant subgaleal or intracranial haemorrhages. Similarly, when neonatal outcomes of vacuum extraction and forceps birth were compared in the review, differences were confined to the clinically nonsignificant effects. Nevertheless, extensive observational data suggest that subgaleal haemorrhage is much more common with vacuum extraction than forceps birth[22] but that the occurrence of intracranial injury is not different between the two methods.[17]

Subgaleal haemorrhage is almost always preceded by difficult vacuum extraction featuring a number of avoidable factors including deflexing and paramedian cup applications, prolonged extractions with excessive number and strength of pulls, cup detachment, often multiple, and failure of the initial vacuum extraction with a subsequent attempt at forceps birth.[23–25]

Effects on the mother

Systematic reviews comparing vacuum extraction and forceps birth have consistently reported more vaginal trauma, anal sphincter damage and genital tract injury with the forceps.[14,26] Damage to the anorectal sphincter muscles during childbirth has long been regarded as a major predisposing factor for the subsequent development of urinary and faecal incontinence[27] yet the evidence to support this is conflicting.[28,29] More recently, there have been a number of reports with data demonstrating a protective effect from vacuum-assisted birth with regard to the later development of urinary and faecal incontinence and pelvic organ prolapse.[30,31] Damage to the sphincter is associated with vacuum extractions that are difficult or that fail, especially if the birth is completed with forceps.[18,19] Therefore, unless operators are appropriately trained in vacuum extraction techniques, the potential advantages for the mother's pelvic floor and perineum may not be fully realised.

Evidence has accumulated showing that liberal use of episiotomy in normal birth does not necessarily prevent severe vaginal or perineal trauma,[14] but the evidence with regard to operative vaginal birth is less clear.[32,33] For vacuum-assisted birth, episiotomy is not routinely required. However, operators should be aware that the perineum of a nulliparous woman may provide significant resistance to birth and, if vacuum extraction is attempted without episiotomy, additional gentle pulls should be provided to allow the perineum to stretch over the advancing fetal head. Recent evidence has demonstrated that midline episiotomy is significantly associated with higher rates of perineal trauma compared with mediolateral episiotomy.[13] It would appear preferable, therefore, to perform mediolateral episiotomy as the method of choice when used in conjunction with vacuum-assisted birth.

Conclusion

Vacuum-assisted birth and its acceptance by clinicians will be determined to a large extent by the number of successful births achieved and by the outcomes for the mother and infant. Clinical audits and system analyses often identify deficient knowledge and inadequate operator training as important contributors to adverse outcomes.[11] The key to avoiding suboptimal outcomes with vacuum-assisted birth is to ensure that the operator's knowledge, skill level and competence are equal to the requirements of the clinical circumstances.[3,34] Training programmes are now available that teach the technique on models that can simulate a realistic vacuum extraction and they should be offered to all obstetric trainees.

References

1. Vacca A. *Handbook of Vacuum Delivery in Obstetric Practice 3rd ed*. Brisbane: Vacca Research; 2009.

2. Vacca A. Vacuum-assisted delivery: An analysis of traction force and maternal and neonatal outcomes. *Aust N Z J Obstet Gynaecol* 2006;46:124–7.

3. *Clinician's Resources for Vacuum Assisted Delivery – Essential Pre-reading for Masterclass in VAD*. (Available at: www.vaccaresearch.com/Free_Clinicians_Resources.htm).

4. Lim FT, Holm JP, Schuitemaker NW, Jansen FH, Hermans J. Stepwise compared with rapid application of vacuum in ventouse extraction procedures. *BJOG* 1997;104:33–6.

5. Bofill JA, Rust OA, Schorr SJ, Brown RC, Roberts WE, Morrison JC. A randomized trial of two vacuum extraction techniques. *Obstet Gynecol* 1997;89:758–62.

6. Muise KL, Duchon MA, Brown RH. Effect of angular traction on the performance of modern vacuum extractors. *Am J Obstet Gynecol* 1992;167:1125–9.

7. O'Neil G. How to get the best results from vacuum extraction. Proceedings from the Sixth Congress of the Federation of the Asia-Oceania Perinatal Societies. 1990;156.

8. Lurie S, Feinstein M, Mamet Y. Assisted internal autorotation with vacuum extractor. Description of an original maneuver. *Arch Obstet Gynecol* 2000;263:93–4.

9. Bird GC. The use of the vacuum extractor. *Clin Obstet Gynaecol* 1982;9:641–61.

10. Lasbrey AH, Orchard CD, Crichton D. A study of the relative merits and scope for vacuum extraction as opposed to forceps delivery. *S Afr J Obstet Gynaecol* 1964;2:1–3.

11. Royal College of Obstetricians and Gynaecologists. *Operative vaginal delivery*. Green-top Guideline No. 26. London: RCOG; 2011.

12. Bird GC. The importance of flexion in vacuum extraction delivery. *Br J Obstet Gynaecol* 1976;83:194–200.

13. American College of Obstetricians and Gynaecologists. *Operative Vaginal Delivery*. ACOG Practice Bulletin No. 17. Washington, DC: ACOG; 2000.

14. O'Mahony F, Hofmeyr GJ, Menon V. Choice of instruments for assisted vaginal delivery. *Cochrane Database Syst Rev* 2010;(11):CD005455.

15. Society of Obstetricians and Gynaecologists of Canada. *Guidelines for Operative Vaginal Birth*. SOGC Clinical Practice Guideline No. 148. Ottawa: SOGC; 2004.

16. O'Driscoll K, Jackson RJA, Gallagher JT. Prevention of prolonged labour. *BMJ* 1969;2:477–80.

17. Towner D, Castro MA, Eby-Wilkins E, Gilbert WM. Effect of mode of delivery in nulliparous women on neonatal intracranial injury. *N Engl J Med* 1999;341:1709–14.

18. Gardella C, Taylor M, Benedetti T, Hitti J, Critchlow C. The effect of sequential use of vacuum and forceps for assisted vaginal delivery on neonatal and maternal outcomes. *Am J Obstet Gynecol* 2001;185:896–902.

19. Demissie K, Rhoads GG, Smulian JC, Balasubramanian BA, Ghandi K, Joseph KS, Kramer M. Operative vaginal delivery and neonatal and infant adverse outcomes: population-based retrospective analysis. *BMJ* 2004;329:1–6.

20. Attilakos G, Sibander T, Winter C, Johnson N, Draycott T. A randomised controlled trial of a new handheld vacuum extraction device. *BJOG* 2005;112:1510–15.

21. Groom KM, Jones BA, Miller N, Paterson-Brown S. A prospective randomised controlled trial of the Kiwi OmniCup versus conventional ventouse cups for vacuum-assisted vaginal delivery. *BJOG* 2006;113:183–9.

22. Chadwick LM, Pemberton PJ, Kurinczuk JJ. Neonatal subgaleal haematoma: Associated risk factors, complications and outcome. *J Paediatr Child Health* 1996;32:228–32.

23. Fortune P-M, Thomas RM. Sub-aponeurotic haemorrhage: a rare but life-threatening neonatal complication associated with ventouse delivery. *BJOG* 1999;106:868–70.

24. Smith SA, Jett PL, Jacobson SL, Binder ND, Kuforiji TA, Gilhooly JT, et al. Subgaleal hematoma: the need for increased awareness of risk. *J Fam Pract* 1995;41:569–74.

25. Ross MG, Fresquez M, El-Haddad MA. Impact of FDA Advisory on reported vacuum-assisted delivery and morbidity. *J Matern Fetal Med* 2000;9:321–6.

26. Eason E, Labrecque M, Wells G, Feldman P. Preventing perineal trauma during childbirth: A systematic review. *Obstet Gynecol* 2000;95:464–71.

27. Mous M, Muller SA, de Leeuw JW. Long-term effects of anal sphincter rupture during vaginal delivery: faecal incontinence and sexual complaints. *BJOG* 2008;115:234–8.

28. Johanson RB, Heycock E, Carter J, Sultan AH, Walklate K, Jones PW. Maternal and child health after assisted vaginal delivery: five-year follow up of a randomised controlled study comparing forceps and ventouse. *BJOG* 1999;106:544–9.

29. Falton DL, Otero M, Petignat P, Sangalli MR, Floris LA, Boulvain M, et al. Women's health 18 years after rupture of the anal sphincter during childbirth: 1. Fecal incontinence. *Am J Obstet Gynecol* 2006;194:1255–99.

30. MacArthur C, Glaxener C, Lancashire R, Herbison P, Wilson D (on behalf of the ProLong study group).Exclusive caesarean section birth and subsequent urinary and faecal incontinence: a 12 year longitudinal study. *BJOG* 2011;118:1001–7.

31. Handa VL, Blomquist JL, McDermott KC, Friedman S, Munoz A. Pelvic floor disorders after vaginal birth: Effect of episiotomy, perineal laceration and operative birth. *Obstet Gynecol* 2012;119:233–9.

32. Murphy DJ, Macleod M, Bahl R, Goyder K, Howarth L, Strachan B. A randomised controlled trial of routine versus restrictive use of episiotomy at operative vaginal delivery: a multicentre pilot study. *BJOG* 2008;115:1695–703.

33. De Leeuw JW, de Wit C, Kuijken JP, Bruinse HW. Mediolateral episiotomy reduces the risk for anal sphincter injury during operative vaginal delivery. *BJOG* 2008;115:104–8.

34. Bahl R, Murphy DJ, Strachan B. Qualitative analysis by interviews and video recordings to establish the components of a skilled low-cavity non-rotational vacuum delivery. *BJOG* 2009;116:319–26.

Chapter 5
Nonrotational forceps and manual rotation

Kim Hinshaw and Shilpa Mahadasu

Key learning points

- Developing skills in nonrotational forceps and manual rotation remains an important element of training in operative obstetrics.
- Active use of simulation is recommended to develop operative vaginal birth skills.
- Forceps are more likely to achieve vaginal birth compared with vacuum extraction but are associated with a higher risk of vaginal and perineal trauma.
- Forceps should be applied with care and correct application to the fetal head should be confirmed before traction is applied.
- Initial traction should be applied using Pajot's manoeuvre, keeping the forceps handles near the horizontal plane until the fetal head is crowning.
- The operator must maintain situational awareness, review whether progress is adequate and be willing to abandon the procedure if necessary.
- Re-assess before proceeding with 'double instrumentation' and involve senior staff if the presenting part is not near the pelvic outlet.
- After forceps birth, always undertake a systematic inspection to exclude maternal trauma.
- Ensure comprehensive record keeping and debrief the mother after birth.

The aim of operative vaginal birth (OVB) is to expedite birth for the benefit of the mother, baby or both while minimising maternal and neonatal morbidity. Worldwide, OVB remains an integral part of the obstetrician's role.[1] Forceps and ventouse are the two instruments used in UK practice, with manual rotation of the fetal head a further option. Historically, obstetric forceps were used at least as early as 1500 BC as both single and paired instruments. Egyptian, Greek, Roman and Persian writing and pictures refer to forceps that were used to extract the dead baby to save the mother's life.[2] In the 16th century, Peter Chamberlen invented the precursors of modern forceps for the birth of live infants. Modifications have led to more than 700 designs with outlet, midcavity and rotational forceps used widely in clinical practice.

Overall, OVB rates in UK have remained fairly constant over the last 35 years, varying between 9% and 14%.[3-5] However, forceps versus vacuum rates vary by country, with rates in 2010 for England at 6.1% versus 6.3%, respectively, whereas in Scotland there is a trend towards increased use of forceps (9.7% versus 2.9%).[4-6] Operative vaginal birth rates in other parts of the world vary from 1.5% of deliveries (Czech Republic) to 15% (Australia and Canada). Other instruments are still used in modern obstetric practice and one example is the 'spatula' used in France. These independent, symmetrical instruments are related to forceps but do not lock together. They are used in pairs to facilitate head descent, with a safety profile and complication rate similar to a standard forceps birth.[7]

A Cochrane review of 32 studies ($n = 6597$) confirmed that forceps were less likely than the vacuum to fail to achieve vaginal birth (relative risk [RR] 0.65, 95% confidence interval [CI] 0.45–0.94) but with significantly more third- or fourth-degree tears, vaginal trauma and rectal incontinence.[8] Facial injury was more likely with forceps (RR 5.10, 95% CI 1.12–23.25) with a trend towards fewer cases of cephalhaematoma with forceps (RR 0.64, 95% CI 0.37–1.11).

There has been a fall in midcavity OVB with operators cautious and perhaps less skilled at undertaking potentially complex forceps/instrumental births. This has resulted in a continuing rise in second-stage caesarean section rates, a potentially difficult procedure associated with higher rates of maternal and neonatal morbidity[9] (see Chapter 7). Direct consultant supervision of obstetric trainees, facilitated by simulation techniques, can accelerate the acquisition of confidence and competence in performing forceps births and these aspects will be discussed later.

The aim of clinical training is to ensure that we produce practitioners who are aware of the correct circumstance in which a particular instrument should be used and who develop appropriate skills in OVB in order to provide women with safe and effective birth.[10] This chapter describes the use of nonrotational forceps in detail and also reviews the technique of manual rotation.

Nonrotational forceps

Nonrotational forceps are mainly used to facilitate vaginal birth when the fetal head is in an occipito-anterior (OA) position. Ideally, the fetal head will lie in the direct OA (DOA) position, but blades can be safely applied when the head lies within 45° of the vertical (i.e. between left OA and right OA positions [Figure 5.1]). Nonrotational forceps may also be used to assist birth in a direct occipito-posterior (DOP) position.

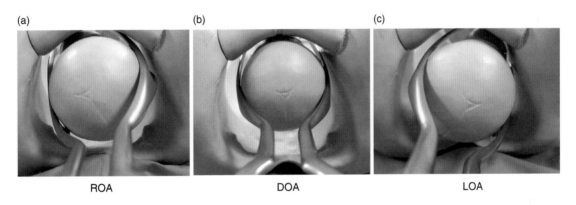

(a)	(b)	(c)
ROA	DOA	LOA

Figure 5.1 Range of positions for safe forceps application

The basic design constitutes a matching pair of forceps blades, nominated left and right relative to where the blade lies when applied within the maternal pelvis. The relevant parts of the forceps are labelled in Figure 5.2.

Forceps are classified according to their design as well as the type of operative birth they are used to perform based on station and position of the fetal head. Several types are in common use in the UK but all are essentially similar in configuration: Simpson, Anderson, Haig-Ferguson, Neville-Barnes and Wrigley's are examples. The choice of forceps is based on individual circumstances and is often subjective. The majority of nonrotational forceps have relatively long handles allowing their use from midcavity or below. Wrigley's forceps have short shanks and handles and are mainly used to assist birth of the head at caesarean section. They may be used as outlet forceps (Figure 5.3).

(a)

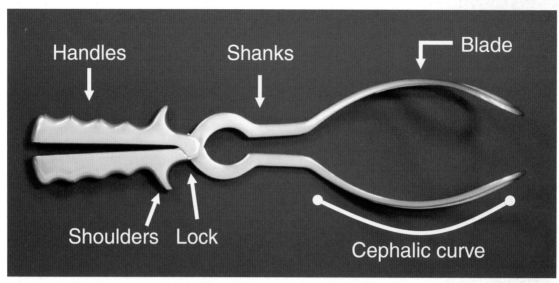

(b)

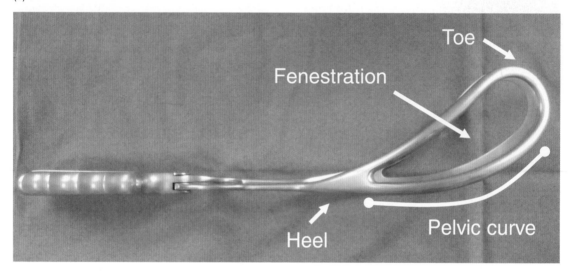

Figure 5.2 Parts of the forceps

Assessment before performing nonrotational forceps

Indications

The indications for considering OVB are discussed in depth in Chapter 2. In the majority of cases, whether for maternal or fetal reasons, the choice between forceps and vacuum depends on the experience of the operator and their assessment of the best instrument to use for the individual circumstances. Nonrotational forceps may be used to facilitate birth from midcavity, low cavity

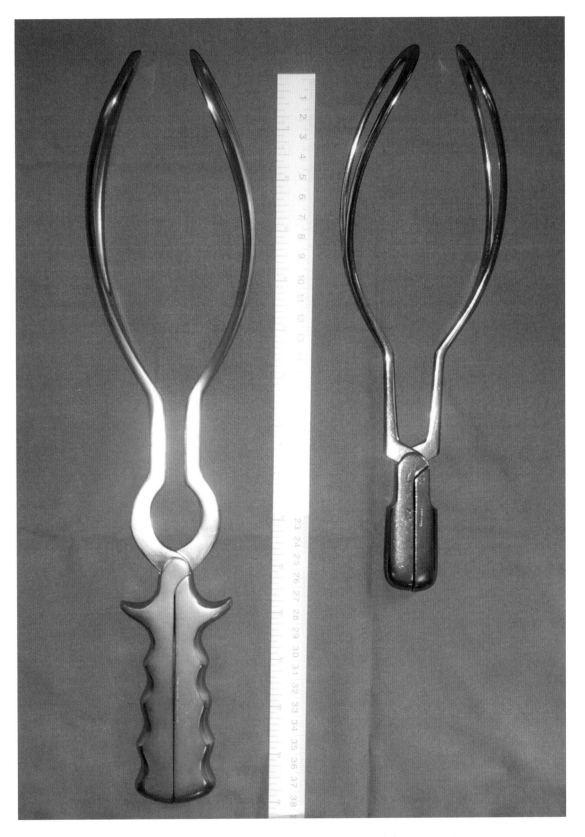

Figure 5.3 Long- and short-handled forceps

or at the pelvic outlet.[10] The most common reasons for OVB are a prolonged second stage and presumed fetal compromise.

Nonrotational forceps should be used in preference to vacuum in certain circumstances:

- face presentation (mento-anterior position)
- assisted birth under 34 weeks.[10]

Nonrotational forceps may be used in preference to vacuum in:

- acute fetal compromise (prolonged bradycardia)
- assisted birth at 34–36 weeks[10]
- midcavity birth OA (particularly a trial in theatre)
- low cavity birth (OP)
- multiple fetal scalp sampling.

Forceps should not be applied before full dilatation of the cervix. One rare relative contraindication is when the fetus is known to have osteogenesis imperfecta, when an individualised decision about mode of birth has to be made after wider discussion.

Clinical and ultrasound assessment

Assessment before undertaking an OVB is discussed in depth in Chapter 2. Careful abdominal and vaginal examination must be performed before undertaking a nonrotational forceps birth. Clinical examination should include consideration of any degree of relative (or absolute) disproportion. A common reason for malpractice litigation is failure to assess the position/level of the fetal head in relation to the pelvic outlet. Most cases of assisted birth where the position is OA are low cavity. Assessment of the position is usually made using the fontanelles and sutures as landmarks. In cases of significant caput, the operator can seek out the pinna of the fetal ear that can only be 'bent' towards the fetal face. Abdominal ultrasound assessment can be a useful adjunct to clinical examination in the second stage and can be used accurately by the novice sonographer.[11,12]

Consent

Verbal consent must be obtained before OVB in the labour room and the discussion documented in the notes. If circumstances allow, written consent should be obtained. Concerns to be covered include the proposed procedure, intended benefits, serious and frequently occurring risks both maternal and fetal (e.g. forceps marks on the baby's face), other procedures that may be required (for forceps birth, episiotomy should be mentioned) and planned analgesia/anaesthesia.[13,14]

Technique for nonrotational forceps

Preparation

Before embarking on a nonrotational forceps birth, the operator should be comfortable and competent to use the selected forceps with the ability to manage any complications that may arise. Adequate supervision must be available if required. Skills lists are available that clearly delineate the steps required to achieve a safe OVB.[15] Having obtained appropriate consent from the woman, the operator should ensure the following factors are also addressed:

- **Team:** A complete team should be available to support the operator. This will vary but may include midwives, a healthcare assistant, a professional trained in neonatal resuscitation, anaesthetist and senior obstetric staff.

- **Analgesia:** Ensure effective analgesia is given. Options for forceps include pudendal block, perineal infiltration, regional blockade and, rarely, general anaesthesia (see Chapter 9).

- **Check instruments:** Check that the equipment is laid out on the trolley in the correct order. Three clamps (two for dividing the cord and one for clamping the cord for cord bloods). Scissors for performing an episiotomy if required. Count the swabs.

- **Positioning:** A modified lithotomy position is best, avoiding excessive hip abduction. The mother should be supported in a semi-upright position and some degree of (left) lateral tilt should be maintained. The buttocks should just protrude beyond the end of the bed.

- **Positioning of the operator:** Operators vary in their preference to sit, stand or kneel while conducting a forceps birth. The operator should be well balanced, predominantly using hands and arms only. Sitting or kneeling may reduce the temptation to use upper bodyweight during traction.

- **Catheterisation:** The operator should scrub up for the procedure before cleansing and draping. The bladder should be catheterised unless this is not possible if the head is very low. If an indwelling catheter is present, either remove the catheter or deflate the balloon during the birth.

Forceps application

■ **Check that the forceps are a correct pair:** All forceps have a number imprinted on them and these should match.

■ **Assembly:** Place the forceps on the trolley 'back to back'. Pick up the left blade with the left hand and right blade with the right hand (Figure 5.4a). To assemble the forceps the blades are crossed, with the right blade lying superior to the left. They meet and join at the 'lock' (Figure 5.4b and 5.4c).

(a)

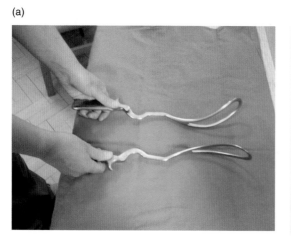

(b)

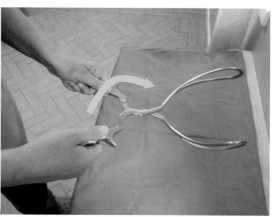

(c)

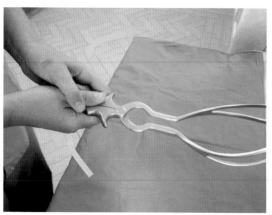

Figure 5.4 Assembling the forceps

■ **Applying the left blade:** The left blade is held between the fingers of the left hand, in a vertical position with a 'light pencil grip'. This grip reminds the operator to avoid using excessive force during insertion. The index and middle fingers of the right hand are inserted through the introitus at the five o'clock position and the tip of the left blade is introduced at that point, keeping the handle vertical and parallel to the patient's right femur. At that point, the inner surface of the forceps blade faces the vulva. The fingers of the right hand protect the maternal soft tissues as the blade is gently inserted to lie in the final position against the left side of the

(a)

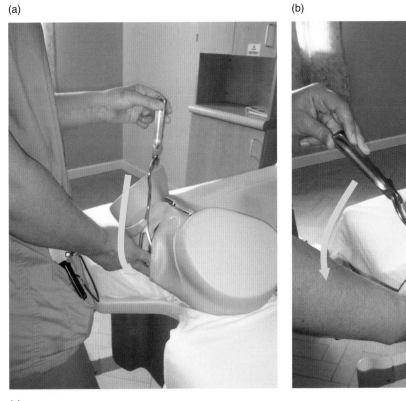

(b)

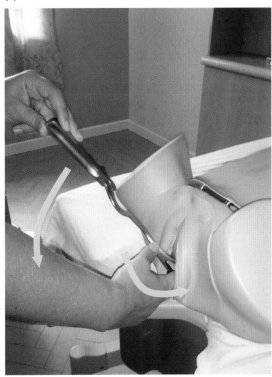

(c)

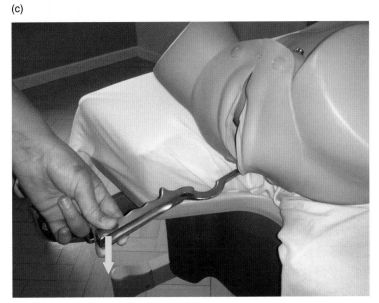

Figure 5.5 Applying the left blade

fetal head. The thumb of the right hand can be placed on the heel of the blade to help insertion. After insertion the handle is pushed gently back against the perineum to hold the blade in position (Figure 5.5a–c).

The right blade is held vertically with the right hand using the same light pencil grip. The index and middle fingers of the left hand are inserted through the introitus at the seven o'clock position. Insertion of both blades should occur easily (Figure 5.6a–c). If insertion proves difficult, remove the blade(s) and carefully re-check the position of the head. Call senior staff if you are unsure.

(a)

(b)

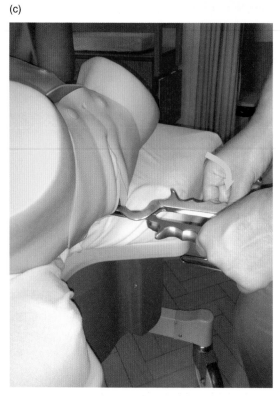
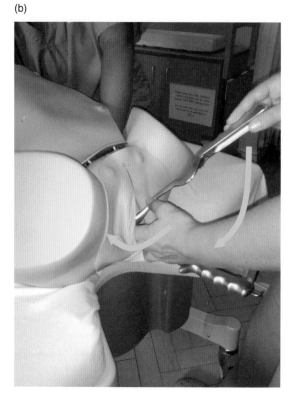

(c)

Figure 5.6 Applying the right blade

(a)

(b)

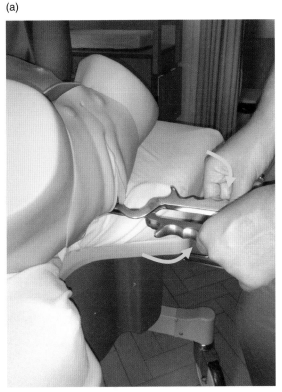
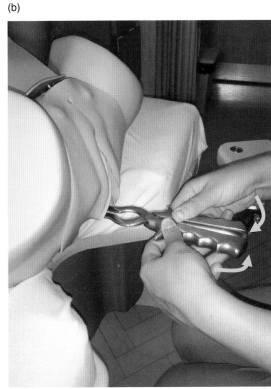

Figure 5.7 Locking the blades

- **Locking the blades:** The left blade is always inserted first, allowing the two forceps blades to be locked without having to 'uncross' the handles. After insertion, the blades may need gentle manipulation in order to get them to 'lock' (Figure 5.7a and 5.7b). Once locked, the operator should avoid holding the handles together as this may lead to compression of the fetal head.

- **Confirming correct application:** Before applying traction, the operator should check that the blades are correctly applied to the fetal head (Figure 5.8a and 5.8b). An index finger can be introduced along the shanks of the forceps to check the following:

  - ☐ the sagittal suture should be central and parallel to the plane of the blades

  - ☐ the lambdoidal sutures should be equidistant from the upper edge of both blades

  - ☐ it should not be possible to introduce more than a fingertip through the fenestration near the heel of the blade (from 'inside to out').

- A well-applied forceps blade should lie along the mento-vertical axis of the fetal skull when the head is OA and well flexed (Figure 5.9). Traction force is mainly applied to the fetal malar bones, accounting for the pressure mark that is often found at that point immediately after birth.

(a)

(b)

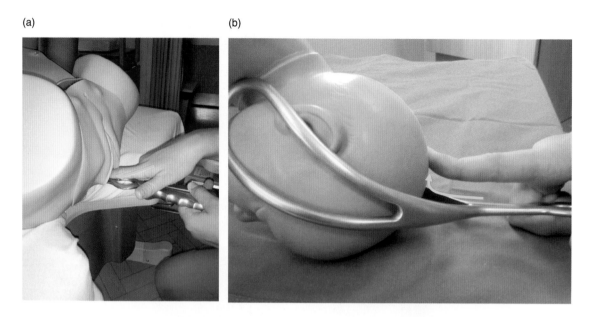

Figure 5.8 Confirming correct application

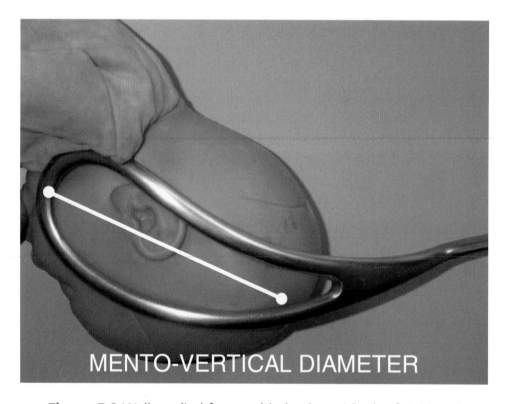

MENTO-VERTICAL DIAMETER

Figure 5.9 Well-applied forceps blade alongside the fetal head

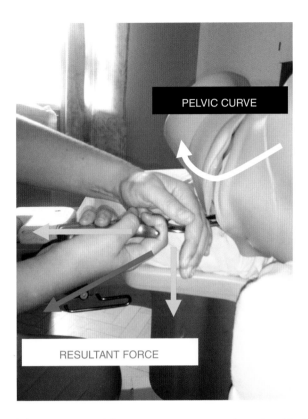

Figure 5.10 The pelvic curve and force vectors associated with Pajot's manoeuvre

Traction

■ **Traction:** Traction should be timed with uterine contractions unless there is acute fetal compromise. Moderate traction using arm and shoulder force only should be adequate. Avoid countertraction against the labour bed with the operator's foot. For midcavity birth, and the initial part of a low cavity birth, the aim is to apply traction along the axis of the mid pelvis. The pelvic curve of the forceps follows the direction of the birth canal and lies along the straight arm of the 'J' shaped pelvic curve.

■ **Pajot's manoeuvre:** Pajot's manoeuvre is used to encourage descent of the fetal head along the straight arm of the pelvic curve. The operator applies horizontal traction force with one hand using the handles/shoulders of the forceps. The other hand applies force vertically downwards over the shanks. These two vector forces must be balanced to produce a resultant vector force that will allow the head to descend along the appropriate path (Figure 5.10).

The forceps handles should be kept more or less horizontal during traction. The most common mistake is to see the forceps handles dropped 30–40° below the horizontal (Figure 5.11a and 5.11b).

The fetal head will gradually descend until the occiput lies under the symphysis pubis.

(a) (b)

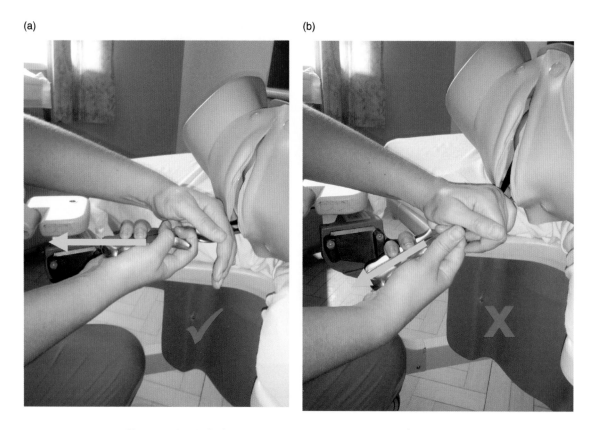

Figure 5.11 Pajot's manoeuvre: correct and incorrect

At that point the operator should stop using Pajot's manoeuvre. The perineum will usually be stretching up against the fetal head as it reaches the pelvic outlet and the need for an episiotomy can be assessed.

- **Episiotomy:** Forceps births are associated with an increased risk of obstetric anal sphincter injury (up to 7%).[16] A retrospective cohort study of 2861 women reported a six-fold decreased odds for developing anal sphincter injury when a mediolateral episiotomy was performed during OVB.[17] Mediolateral episiotomy directed laterally at an angle of at least 60° in the direction of ischial tuberosity resulted in a low incidence of anal sphincter tearing, anal incontinence and perineal pain (Figure 5.12).[8,18] RCOG guidance recommends restrictive use of episiotomy in OVB, using the operator's individual judgment in each case.[10]

- **Completing delivery of the head:** The handles of the forceps are brought up in a gentle curve using one hand, while the other hand guards the perineum to reduce the risk of significant perineal trauma. By the time the head is completely delivered, the forceps handles will be vertical over the symphysis pubis (Figure 5.13).

- **Removing the forceps:** The forceps blades should be carefully 'unlocked' and removed by sliding them gently off the head (Figure 5.14a and 5.14b).

(a)

(b)

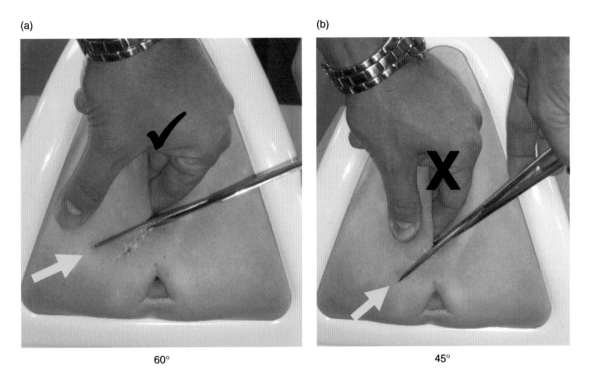

60°   45°

Figure 5.12 Appropriate angle for episiotomy

(a)

(b)

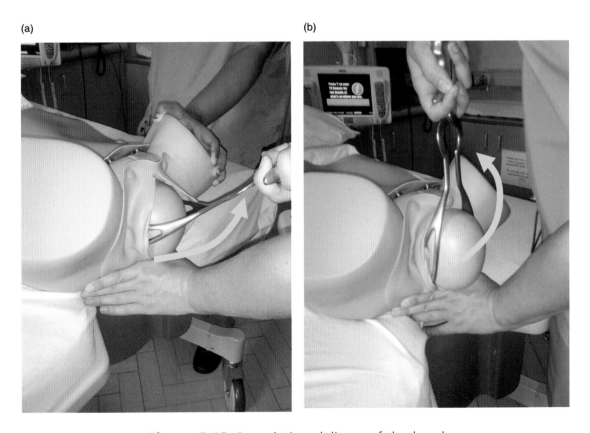

Figure 5.13 Completing delivery of the head

(a)

(b)

(c)

(d)

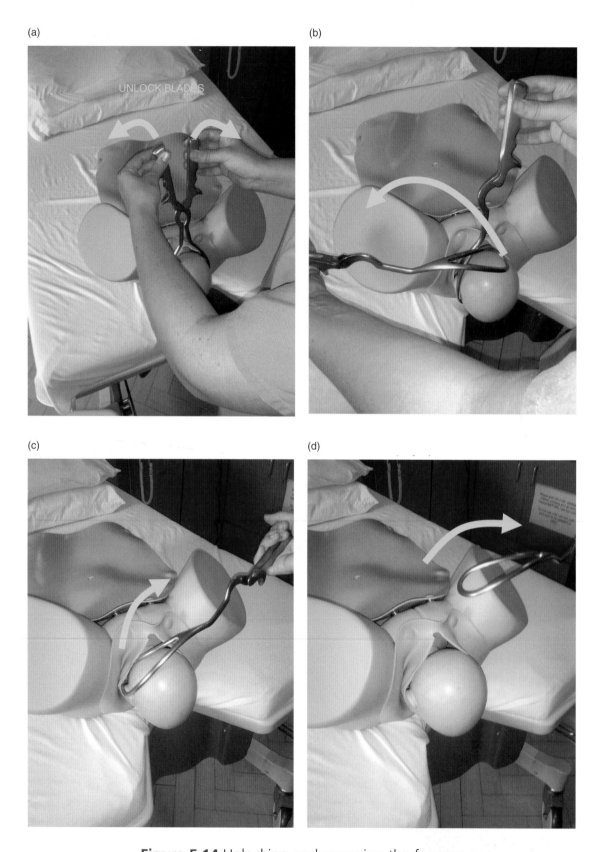

Figure 5.14 Unlocking and removing the forceps

■ **Completing the birth:** This mirrors the process of normal birth. Be aware of the increased risk of shoulder dystocia. In the absence of fetal compromise, ask the mother if she would like the baby placed on her abdomen. The third stage should be actively managed. Ensure the placenta is complete.

■ **Assessing for trauma post-birth:** The genital tract should be inspected systematically to detect trauma and repair undertaken.

Record keeping and debriefing the woman

After every OVB the operator must ensure that a comprehensive, accurate and contemporaneous record is made, which is signed and dated appropriately. This will include details of prior assessment, the procedure itself and the initial condition of the baby (including Apgar scores and cord pH as per local protocols). Specific detail on the number of pulls, number of contractions, traction force, etc. should be noted. Completion of the third stage of labour, assessment for trauma and consequent repair, swab and instrument count and estimated blood loss should also be recorded. Electronic records for OVB can enhance the amount of detail recorded for future reference. The RCOG guidance on OVB includes an example record sheet in the appendices.[10] The record should also give clear and specific instructions for postbirth care: bladder drainage, analgesic requirements, VTE prophylaxis, perineal care, etc.

Follow up of the mother can be difficult because of early discharge policies and out of hours rota systems. However, it is vital that the operator aims to visit the mother before discharge home for a short, focused debrief. This will allow discussion about any questions or concerns that the mother may have. Women can be reassured that the risk of a forceps in future pregnancies is usually very low. All obstetricians should consider using a validated tool to assess patient perception of the OVB. The SaFE Patient Perception Score (PPS) is simple for patients to complete with high internal reliability.[19] Direct patient assessment of clinical practice can facilitate learning and appraisal. Low scores are infrequent but can be used to address concerns for individual operators. Women tend to highlight concerns about 'nontechnical' rather than 'technical skills', which include matters related to decision making, communication, etc. (see Chapter 3).

Manual rotation

An alternative to vacuum rotation is manual rotation from OT or OP positions. After successful rotation, birth may be spontaneous or assisted

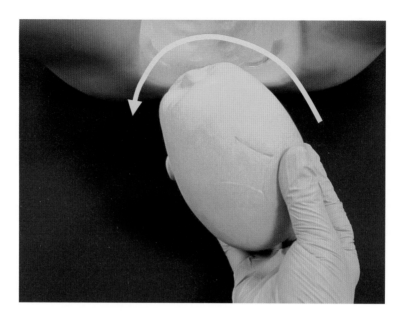

Figure 5.15 Manual rotation

(using forceps or vacuum). There is evidence that manual/digital rotation from a posterior to anterior position may reduce the number of OVBs[20,21] and caesarean sections.[21]

The techniques described vary. The simplest involves encouraging rotation of the head from the transverse towards an OA position by applying pressure on the lambdoidal suture of the fetal head during a contraction, aided by maternal effort. This may lead to spontaneous birth or an OVB.

The technique of formal manual rotation for persistent OP position involves placing the whole of the operator's hand within the vagina to lie in the lower pelvis behind the fetal head. The hand acts as a 'surrogate' for the gutter formed by the pelvic floor muscles. For a left OP position, the right hand is inserted (vice versa for a right OP position). This requires gentle insertion and adequate analgesia should be in place. For a multiparous woman, use of entonox may be appropriate, but pudendal or regional blockade will usually be required for nulliparous women. The thumb is then positioned alongside the anterior fontanelle (Figure 5.15). The mother is asked to push with a contraction and the operator applies pressure with the thumb to flex the head. As flexion occurs, the head will start to rotate towards an OA position with minimal effort from the operator. When rotation has been achieved, the mother can be asked to push with the aim of completing the birth herself. If descent does not occur (or if fetal condition requires intervention), the operator can proceed to an OVB. Note: the fetal head is not disimpacted when using this technique for manual rotation.

Special circumstances

Traction and birth in low OP position

If the head remains in a DOP position and is low cavity (2 cm or more below the ischial spines), the option of nonrotational forceps can be considered (i.e. 'face to pubes'). However, completing the birth in this position requires downwards traction to be maintained for longer and a large episiotomy is usually required. The deflexed occiput predisposes to an increased risk of third or fourth degree tear. There may be advantages to undertaking a vacuum-assisted birth as rotation to OA position can occur even on the perineum. Midcavity OP positions should ideally be rotated using vacuum, Kielland's or manual rotation.

Face presentation

Nonrotational forceps may be used when there is a need to expedite birth in the second stage. This only applies to a face presentation in the mento-anterior position. The forceps technique is similar to that outlined above for OP birth.

Abandoning a procedure and use of sequential instruments

In undertaking a forceps birth, the operator must ensure that adequate progress is being made throughout the operative birth process. Maintaining a 'willingness to abandon' the procedure is vital to ensure the safety of both mother and neonate. In particular, the operator must avoid using increased traction force or too many pulls when there is failure of descent. The RCOG recommends that procedures should be abandoned where there is no evidence of progressive descent with moderate traction during each contraction, or where birth is not imminent following three contractions of a correctly applied instrument by an experienced operator.[10]

At times, the first instrument may fail and the situation should be critically reviewed before a second instrument is applied. Vacuum-assisted birth has a higher failure rate than forceps and the second instrument used in most sequential attempts at vaginal birth is forceps.[8,22] The decision to abandon the procedure after use of one instrument has to be balanced with the risks of a full dilatation caesarean section with increased maternal and neonatal morbidity.[9,10,22–26] There is clearly a difference between completion of the birth using a second instrument from the level of the pelvic outlet and use of a second instrument following a failed attempt at midcavity rotation. One example to consider would be a vacuum undertaken for delay associated with a transverse position. If there has been good descent and rotation, but the vacuum cup 'pops off' a couple of times on or near the perineum, it would be reasonable to complete the birth with low-cavity, nonrotational forceps (after carefully re-assessing the position). A cohort study of 1360 nulliparous women concluded that the use of sequential instruments was associated with greater maternal and neonatal morbidity compared with forceps alone (anal sphincter tear odds ratio [OR] 1.8, 95% CI 1.1–2.9; umbilical artery pH <7.10 OR 3.0, 95% CI 1.7–5.5).[25] Intracranial haemorrhage occurs in 1 in 256 births following sequential instrumentation compared with 1 in 334 for failed forceps proceeding to caesarean section.[10] Improved training in decision making, clinical assessment and appropriate selection and use of instruments is required, to ensure that we maximise the rate of completing the birth with one instrument. The majority of cases where use of a second instrument is planned should be discussed with a consultant before proceeding.

Trial of OVB in theatre

The RCOG recommends that OVBs that have a higher risk of failure should be considered a trial and conducted in a place where immediate recourse to caesarean section can be undertaken.[10] Factors that are associated with higher failure rates are maternal body mass index (BMI) >30, estimated fetal weight >4000 g or clinically big baby, OP position and midcavity birth or when one-fifth of the head is palpable per abdomen. The incidence of trial of OVB is estimated at 2–5%.[27] The most common reason for a 'trial in theatre' is to manage arrested progress in the second stage of labour at midcavity, which may be attributable to relative cephalopelvic disproportion (CPD), with immediate resort to caesarean section if needed.[28] Moving to theatre is associated with a longer decision to delivery interval (DDI) compared with OVB in the labour room (mean [SD] 14.5 [9.5] vs. 30.0 [14.6] minutes) but this is not associated with any increase in neonatal morbidity.[29] One problem associated with a trial in theatre is the potential loss of maternal assistance related to use of dense spinal/epidural blockade, often inserted in preparation for a possible caesarean section. This problem may be compounded by the use of vacuum techniques and consequently higher failure rates.[8] For a trial where rotation is not required, particularly when the level is midcavity (ischial spines 0–2 cm below), the practitioner should consider using nonrotational forceps as the instrument of choice to maximise the potential for successful vaginal birth. Unfortunately, at present there is no current evidence from randomised trials to influence practice.[27]

Consultant presence and supervision

Forceps birth requires competence and confidence, both of which are acquired by practical experience. With reduced training time, trainees may be reluctant to attempt what they perceive as difficult procedures if the consultant is not on the labour ward.[30] The RCOG recommends that 'an experienced operator, competent at mid-cavity deliveries, should be present from the outset for all attempts at rotational or mid-cavity operative vaginal delivery'.[10] In many circumstances this will require the presence of the consultant. Murphy et al.[31] concluded that senior operators were less likely to proceed to caesarean section and there was less likelihood of major haemorrhage (OR 0.5, 95% CI 0.3–0.9). The same study noted an increase in maternal and neonatal morbidity associated with birth by second-stage caesarean section. In previous work, Murphy et al. noted that operator inexperience led to excessive pulls and use of multiple instruments that could be addressed by consultant input in both decision making and the conduct of complex operative vaginal births.[28] In a small observational study ($n = 32$), Oláh[32] confirmed that when a registrar decision to proceed directly to lower segment caesarean section in the second stage was followed by a consultant examination within 15 minutes, the decision was reversed and successful operative vaginal birth achieved in 63% of cases. Another small cohort study ($n = 50$) confirmed that consultant presence for trials in theatre significantly increased vaginal birth rates (70% [7/10] vs 30% [12/40]; $P < 0.05$).[30] Direct consultant input in more complex forceps births (eg trials in theatre) is an invaluable training opportunity, allowing immediate feedback for the trainee and improvement in clinical technique. Second-stage caesarean section rates remain a cause for concern[33] and may be reduced by consultant presence. Larger studies are required to confirm the true effect/benefit of increased consultant presence and supervision in the conduct of forceps birth.

The role of simulation in training

Simulation in obstetrics allows training and practice in a safe environment and can improve the performance of individuals and obstetric teams. There is overwhelming evidence that simulated practice leads to improvement for obstetricians in both their technical and communication skills.[34] Traditionally, practical obstetric skills have been learned by observation followed by direct supervision on patients. Patient safety is another driver for increased use of simulation in training for forceps birth. Use of pelvic mannequins is not new and was actively promoted in the 18th century by the French midwife Madame Du Coudray. Simple mannequins allow the trainee to develop both technical skills and a systematic approach to forceps birth. They allow trainees to build confidence and trainers can objectively assess trainees' progress. There are an increasing number of more sophisticated simulators: Dupuis et al.[35] have developed a spatial tracking system that assesses the trajectory of the forceps blade during application in a childbirth simulator. Objective assessment of traction force during simulation training for shoulder dystocia demonstrated a reduction in applied traction force after training.[36] Subsequent studies confirmed a reduction in brachial plexus injury in hospitals that had undertaken the training programme. Objective assessments of traction force and the vector of the force on the baby during normal and operative vaginal birth have recently been described using the 'Peisner Platform'. The maximum pulling force exerted on the fetus ranged from 31.7 N to135.4 N (7lb 2oz to 30lb 7oz) over 8 to 51 seconds.[37]

In all of the above, simulation focuses on two main aspects of forceps birth that need to be mastered, namely forceps application and traction skills. Other areas of simulation training concentrate on the important area of 'nontechnical skills', which is also relevant to undertaking a forceps birth (e.g. situational awareness, decision making, task management, team working and communication, etc.).[38] Simulation is an adjunct to clinical exposure but is an important step in ensuring better training in the use of forceps.

Summary

Nonrotational forceps remains an important component of the skill set that the obstetrician should be able to offer women. A skilled practitioner will be aware of the correct clinical situation in which forceps may give maximum benefit to mother and baby. Midcavity forceps skills require supervised training at senior level if this option is to be maintained and the rising rate of second-stage caesarean section addressed. Manual rotation is an alternative skill that practitioners should learn and may be particularly of benefit to multiparous women with a malposition. Simulation has a vital role in developing and maintaining forceps skills and should include training in both 'technical' and 'nontechnical' skills.

References

1. Hillier CE, Johansson RB. Worldwide survey of operative vaginal delivery. *Int J Gynaecol Obstet* 1994;47:109–14.

2. Ross MG, Forceps Delivery [emedicine.medscape.com/article/263603-overview].

3. Royal College of Obstetricians and Gynaecologists Clinical Effectiveness Support Unit. *The National Sentinel Caesarean Section Audit Report*. London: RCOG Press, 2001.

4. Birth choice UK Maternity statistics (1976–2011) [http://www.birthchoiceuk.com/Professionals/index.html].

5. Births in Scottish Hospitals. *Information Services Division*, NHS Scotland, 30 August 2011 [http://www.isdscotland.org/Health-Topics/Maternity-and-Births/Publications/2011–08–30/2011–08–30-Births-Report.pdf].

6. NHS *Maternity statistics, England 2010–11*. The Information Centre for Health and Social Care. 1 December 2011 [https://catalogue.ic.nhs.uk/publications/hospital/maternity/nhs-mater-eng-2010–2011/nhs-mate-eng-2010–2011-pra.pdf].

7. Boucoiran I, Valerio L, Bafghi A, Delotte J, Bongain A. Spatula-assisted deliveries: a large cohort of 1065 cases. *Eur J Obstet Gynecol Reprod Biol* 2010;151:46–51.

8. O'Mahony F, Hofmeyr GJ, Menon V. Choice of instruments for assisted vaginal delivery. *Cochrane Database Syst Rev* 2010;(11):CD005455.

9. Alexander JM, Leveno KJ, Rouse DJ, Landon MB, Gilbert S, Spong CY, et al. Comparison of maternal and infant outcomes from primary cesarean delivery during the second compared with first stage of labor. *Obstet Gynecol* 2007;109:917–21.

10. Royal College of Obstetricians and Gynaecologists. *Operative vaginal delivery*. Green-top Guideline No. 26. London: RCOG; 2011.

11. Yeo L, Romero R. Sonographic evaluation in the second stage of labour to improve the assessment of labor progress and its outcome. *Ultrasound Obstet Gynecol* 2009;33:253–8.

12. Ramphul M, Kennelly M, Murphy DJ. Establishing the accuracy and acceptability of abdominal ultrasound to define the foetal head position in the second stage of labour: a validation study. *Eur J Obstet Gynecol Reprod Biol* 2012;164:35–9.

13. Royal College of Obstetrics and Gynaecologists. *Operative vaginal delivery*. Consent Advice No.11. London: RCOG; 2010.

14. Royal College of Obstetricians and Gynaecologists. *Obtaining valid consent*. Clinical Governance Advice No. 6. London: RCOG; 2008.

15. Bahl R, Murphy DJ, Strachan B. Qualitative analysis by interviews and video recordings to establish the components of a skilled low-cavity non-rotational vacuum delivery. *BJOG* 2009;116:319–26.

16. Fernando RJ, Williams AA, Adams EJ. *The management of third- and fourth-degree perineal tears*. Green-top Guideline No. 29. London: RCOG; 2007.

17. de Vogel J, Van der Leeuw-van Beek A, Gietelink D, Vujkovic M, de Leeuw JW, van Bavel J, et al. The effect of a mediolateral episiotomy during operative vaginal delivery on the risk of developing obstetrical anal sphincter injuries. *Am J Obstet Gynecol* 2012;206:404. e1–5.

18. Kalis V, Landsmanova J, Bednarova B, Karbanova J, Laine K, Rokyta Z. Evaluation of the incision angle of mediolateral episiotomy at 60 degrees. *Int J Gynaecol Obstet* 2011;112:220–4.

19. Siassakos D, Clark J, Sibanda T, Attilakos G, Jefferys A, Cullen L, Bisson D, Draycott T. A simple tool to measure patient perceptions of operative birth. *BJOG* 2009;116:1755–61.

20. Vayssie C, Beucher G, Dupuis O, Feraud O, Simon-Toulza C, Sentilhes L, et al. Instrumental delivery: clinical practice guidelines from the French College of Gynaecologists and Obstetricians. *Eur J Obstet Gynecol Reprod Biol* 2011;159:43–8.

21. Reichman O, Gdansky E, Latinsky B, Labi S, Samueloff A. Digital rotation from occipito-posterior to occipito-anterior decreases the need for caesarean section. *Eur J Obstet Gynecol Reprod Biol* 2008;136:25–8.

22. Sikolia ZW, Achila B, Gudu N. Factors contributing to failure of vacuum delivery and associated maternal/neonatal morbidity. *Int J Gynecol Obstet* 2011;115:157–60.

23. Gardella C, Taylor M, Benedetti T, Hitti J, Critchlow C. The effect of sequential use of vacuum and forceps for assisted vaginal delivery on neonatal and maternal outcomes. *Am J Obstet Gynecol* 2001;185:896–902.

24. Al-Kadri H, Sabr Y, Al-Saif S, Abulaimoun B, Ba'Aqeel H, Saleh A. Failed individual and sequential instrumental vaginal delivery: contributing risk factors and maternal-neonatal complications. *Acta Obstet Gynecol Scand* 2003;82:642–8.

25. Murphy DJ, Macleod M, Bahl R, Strachan B. A cohort study of maternal and neonatal morbidity in relation to use of sequential instruments at operative vaginal delivery. *Eur J Obstet Gynecol Reprod Biol* 2011;156:41–5.

26. Barata S, Cardoso E, Ferreira Santo S, Clode N, Mendes, Graça L. Maternal and neonatal immediate effects of sequential delivery. *J Matern Fetal Neonatal Med* 2012;25:981–3.

27. Majoko F, Gardener G. Trial of instrumental delivery in theatre versus immediate caesarean section for anticipated difficult assisted births. *Cochrane Database Syst Rev* 2012;(10): CD005545.

28. Murphy DJ, Liebling RE, Patel R, Verity L, Swingler R. Cohort study of operative delivery in the second stage of labour and standard of obstetric care. *BJOG* 2003;110:610–15.

29. Murphy DJ, Koh DKM. Cohort study of the decision to delivery interval and neonatal outcome for emergency operative vaginal delivery. *Am J Obstet Gynecol* 2007;196:145.e1–145.e7.

30. Lewis EA, Barr C, Thomas K. The mode of delivery in women taken to theatre at full dilatation: does consultant presence make a difference? *J Obstet Gynaecol* 2011;31:229–31.

31. Murphy DJ, Liebling RE, Verity L, Swingler R, Patel R. Early maternal and neonatal morbidity associated with operative delivery in second stage of labour: a cohort study. *Lancet* 2001;358:1203–7.

32. Oláh KS. Reversal of the decision for caesarean section in the second stage of labour on the basis of consultant vaginal assessment. *J Obstet Gynaecol* 2005;25:115–16.

33. Unterscheider J, McMenamin M, Cullinane F. Rising rates of caesarean deliveries at full cervical dilatation: a concerning trend. *Europ J Obstet Gynecol Reprod Biol* 2011;157:141–4.

34. Argani CH, Eichelberger M, Deering S, Satin AJ. The case for simulation as part of a comprehensive patient safety program. *Am J Obstet Gynecol* 2012;206:451–5.

35. Dupuis O, Decullier E, Clerc J, Moreau R, Pham MT, Bin-Dorel S, et al. Does forceps training on a birth simulator allow obstetricians to improve forceps blade placement? *Eur J Obstet Gynecol Reprod Biol* 2011;159:305–9.

36. Crofts JF, Bartlett C, Ellis D, Hunt LP, Fox R, Draycott TJ. Training for shoulder dystocia: a trial of simulation using low-fidelity and high-fidelity mannequins. *Obstet Gynecol* 2006;108:1477–85.

37. Peisner DB. A device that measures the pulling force and vector of delivering a baby. *Am J Obstet Gynecol* 2011;205:221 e1–7.

38. Bahl R, Murphy DJ, Strachan B. Non-technical skills for obstetricians conducting forceps and vacuum deliveries: qualitative analysis by interviews and video recordings. *Eur J Obstet Gynecol Reprod Biol* 2010;150:147–51.

Chapter 6
Rotational forceps

Karl SJ Oláh

Key learning points

■ Rotational forceps are an instrument that every labour ward specialist should be experienced with.

■ Know, do not guess, the fetal position and station prior to any operative birth.

■ Choose the instrument for birth most appropriate for the circumstances: be familiar with all instruments, not just one.

■ Rotational (Kielland's) forceps are the instrument par excellence for the occipito-posterior (OP) position.

■ Rotational forceps should be conducted in theatre, usually under spinal or epidural anaesthesia.

■ The use of rotational forceps requires a tactile sensory input through the instrument; they are not to be used with force.

■ The angle of traction must follow the angle of the birth canal, which, in view of the lack of pelvic curve on the instrument, is more acute (a more downward pull towards the floor) than that used with traction forceps.

■ Do not force any stage of the procedure (application of blades, rotation). Do not be afraid to abandon the procedure and perform a caesarean section.

In 1915, Christian Kielland (1871–1941) first described his forceps to achieve birth from the midpelvis in cases of malrotation (OP and occipito-transverse [OT] positions of the fetal head).[1,2] Kielland (sometimes spelt Kjelland) described his forceps to be applied for a condition that would not be applicable today (the fetal head arrested in a high transerve or OP position), and in a manner which would be considered dangerous in modern practice. However, the instrument was adopted and adapted and became popular for use by obstetricians in cases of malposition for many years.

Most of the studies of Kielland's forceps, with the exception of some minor studies,[3] do not show any significant excess of fetal or maternal complications as a result of their use.[4–7] A lot of the concern arose in the 1980s when there were a few high-profile medico-legal cases, and there was a lot of optimism that the ventouse would do the same job but with fewer adverse effects. Indeed, the suggestion to consign the instrument to the obstetric museum was first made then, and the final death knell was sounded by the studies comparing it unfavourably with the ventouse.[8,9] A recognised disadvantage of the ventouse is its higher rate of failure to achieve a vaginal birth compared with forceps.[7] The failures occur in three groups: women with large babies, prolonged second stage of labour and OP position.[10] More recently, Kielland's forceps have been shown to be associated with a high success rate in terms of birth (failure to effect birth is approximately 10% in most series) and an apparently low maternal and neonatal morbidity.[11] The data support the continued use of this instrument in selected cases using the expertise of a senior obstetrician.

There has been recent concern about the increasing number of caesarean sections that are being performed in the second stage of labour, and some evidence that this may be, at least in part, due to a 'de-skilling' in the art of operative vaginal birth, in particular the knowledge and use of forceps.[12–15] While rates of successful operative vaginal birth are decreasing, recent attempts at reducing caesarean section rates have highlighted a need for further training in operative vaginal birth.[12] Part of this modern impetus to arm our future obstetricians with the tools required to undertake successful operative vaginal births must also involve the use of rotational or Kielland's forceps, as it is the instrument of choice in the OP position.[11]

Malposition

Transverse position and transverse arrest

True 'deep transverse arrest', which is associated with CPD, is rare. Most cases in which the fetus is found to be in a transverse position are attributable to a failure to rotate, generally as a result of an epidural block that has altered the muscular component of the rotational mechanism. Kielland's original application of the forceps to a fetus in a transverse position was probably because they were applied to a high head that had not yet had a chance to undergo rotation in the midpelvis. True transverse arrest will be associated with caput, moulding and asynclitism.

Asynclitism

Asynclitism is the oblique presentation of the fetal head in labour, and is important in the context of Kielland's forceps as it is corrected by the sliding lock on the instrument. Asynclitism may result from dystocia rather than being the cause of it and a comprehensive understanding of the process is required. As a result of asynclitism in a transverse arrest, either the anterior or the posterior parietal bone presents.

In anterior parietal presentation (Naegele's obliquity), the posteriorly lying parietal bone is arrested by the promontory of the sacrum (Figure 6.1). In the posterior parietal bone presentation (Litzmann's obliquity), the anterior parietal bone is arrested at the symphysis while the posterior parietal bone engages in the brim (Figure 6.2). This latter situation is often considered less favourable than the former.[16]

Occipito-posterior position

The appropriate management of the baby in an OP position remains one of the major challenges to the modern obstetrician. When birth is delayed in the second stage, the best mode of birth may be with Kielland's forceps. The use

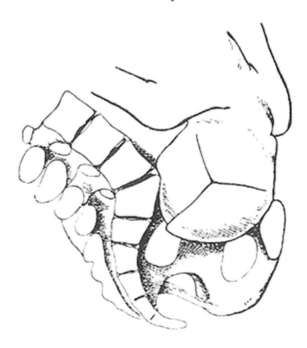

Figure 6.1 Anterior parietal presentation (Naegele's obliquity)

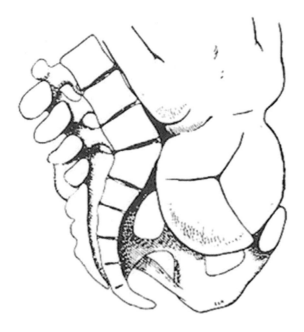

Figure 6.2 Posterior parietal presentation (Litzmann's obliquity)

of the ventouse is more likely to result in failure, requiring a caesarean section.[10] Using traction forceps to bring the baby out 'face to pubes' is more likely to result in trauma and increases the fetal and maternal morbidity. It has been recognised for many years that where the baby is bought out 'face to pubes' the amount of trauma to the mother and baby is often excessive, with an increased incidence of third- and fourth-degree tears. It is well known that the dimensions at the pelvic outlet required for birth in an OP position are greater as the fetal head cannot flex and then extend around the symphysis as it does in an occipito-anterior (OA) position.

Kielland's forceps – an instrument for modern obstetric practice

The modern obstetrician should be able to assess a clinical situation and then decide which instrument is best suited to effect a safe birth. While in most cases the ventouse would be the best instrument to use, or occasionally traction forceps, rotational forceps have a place for those deliveries that require definitive rotation. They should be considered the instrument of choice in OP position of the fetal head, and may be a useful tool where there is a transverse position and a suspicion of true deep transverse arrest. Essentially, a good practitioner should have access to and experience of all these instruments. Inability to use Kielland's forceps deprives the accoucheur of a tool *par excellence* for birth of a baby in an OP position. As an analogy, a mechanic may consider that the best tool to remove a bolt is a spanner. If the mechanic cannot use a spanner because of lack of experience or training, the mechanic may consider using a large wrench instead. The bolt may not come out with the wrench as it may slip off, and if it does, the bolt may be damaged by the use of a nonprecision tool.

General features of the forceps

The measurements of the forceps are not important. However, the features of the instrument (Figure 6.3) that are important are:

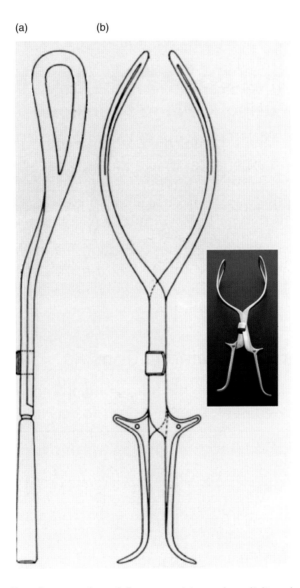

Figure 6.3 Kielland's rotational forceps. Note the sliding lock (a) and the lack of a pelvic curve (b). The blades are fenestrated to reduce the weight of the instrument.

■ The sliding lock. This makes the instrument unique in it is ability to correct asynclitism associated with obstructed labour.

■ The absence of any appreciable pelvic curve. This means that when the forceps are rotated about their axis, the ends of the blades do not describe a circle, they rotate around their axis. Trying the same thing with Simpson's or Neville Barnes forceps results in a large circular motion of the forceps tips.

■ The direction indicator markers. These are small nodular metal markings on the shanks or handles that indicate which way the occiput should be in relation to the forceps.

The forceps themselves are light, with fenestrated blades and with handles that, if compressed, will approximate the blades.

Who should be using Kielland's forceps?

It is essential that Kielland's forceps are used only by obstetricians with the necessary training and experience. Unlike the ventouse, which unfortunately is sometimes used without the position of the fetal head being known with certainty, with Kielland's forceps the position of the fetal head must be known precisely. In addition, because the Kielland's forceps require experience and some degree of sensitivity and feedback through the instrument with regard to tissue resistance, it is expected that use of the Kielland's forceps would take place once a trainee has had some experience with the traction forceps.

Prerequisites and contraindications

For a safe Kielland's forceps birth, the rules that apply to any operative vaginal birth should be followed (see Chapter 2).[16,17] The cervix should be fully dilated. The head should be engaged. The position and station of the head must be known. There must be a valid reason to perform the OVB (usually failure to progress in the second stage of labour). Where there is suspected fetal compromise, an assessment of the severity of that must be made first. If severe (eg bradycardia) it is safer to proceed to caesarean section in most cases. Where there is a 'suspicious' CTG the birth may proceed, or a fetal blood sample may be taken if the CTG is pathological to ensure good fetal reserve prior to continuing with the birth.

The woman should be informed of the reasons for the OVB and, if there is a possibility that the birth may not be successful, the consent for such must be obtained. The anaesthetist must be made aware of the possibility of a caesarean birth and a multidisciplinary approach should always be followed.

Kielland's forceps births should be conducted in theatre with good analgesia, which means a spinal or topped-up epidural block. The use of a pudendal block will probably not be adequate for most cases, and once the birth has commenced it is difficult to then stop and consider such action.

The woman should be placed in lithotomy. A clean operative field should be established as much as possible. The bladder should always be emptied. Finally, a thorough vaginal examination is performed to establish the findings.

Vaginal examination and preparation for application of forceps

It may seem de rigeur to perform a vaginal examination before an OVB. However, it has been reported that the findings of vaginal examinations performed by trainees suggest either a lack of avidity in establishing the fetal position, or a bias in the vaginal assessment findings to try to avoid an OVB in favour of a caesarean section.[14] When performing a vaginal examination before a Kielland's forceps birth it is important to try to get it right.

Always document all the features of the vaginal findings, including the dilatation, the fetal station, the degree of moulding, caput and any other features that may be relevant, such as prominence of the ischial spines or narrowness of the subpubic arch. Also note whether there is a lot of space around the fetal head in the pelvis. Note any asynclitism, and try and establish whether it is an anterior or posterior parietal bone presentation. Finally, and most importantly, the position needs to be established. Using the occiput as the denominator, describe the position as LOT/LOP/Direct OP/ROT or ROT. If there is caput, feel for the fontanelles and suture lines. Remember that the back of the parietal bones have a serrated surface. Also, where there is continuing doubt, feel for the ears of the fetus. Where there is marked deflexion make sure that you feel for a nose or eye sockets in case it is a brow presentation.

Some obstetricians prefer to check the fetal position by ultrasound. While this might be an accurate way to check the fetal position, it in no way should replace the vaginal examination. Those that advocate the use of ultrasound should make a full assessment digitally first, and check their findings ultrasonically if they desire. There is so much more that can be gleaned from a digital examination than from ultrasonic imaging alone.

Once the position is identified, and you are happy that a Kielland's forceps birth is the most appropriate birth, you are ready to apply the forceps. Take the forceps and assemble them in front of the perineum. Remember that the small buttons on the shanks of the forceps indicate where the occiput should be. Therefore, assemble them with the small buttons pointing towards the occiput. Finally, lubricate the forceps with obstetric cream and prepare to apply the blades.

Application

General

The forceps should be held with a light grip, and not clenched with the intention of rotating the fetal head come what may. Parry-Jones,[18] in his book on the subject, suggested using the tips of the fingers, and there is much to commend this approach.

Transverse position

With a fetus in the transverse position there are two options for forceps application:

- **Direct application.** The anterior blade is applied first. The blade is positioned with the direction indicator knob pointing towards the occiput, and the blade passed over the fetal head in a similar way to that which is used when applying traction forceps posteriorly (Figure 6.4). Once the

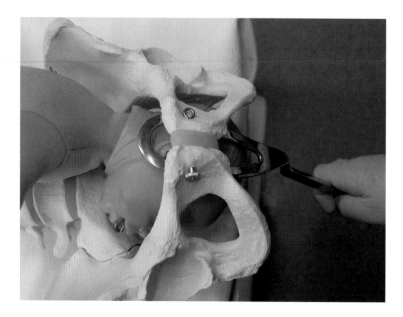

Figure 6.4 Transverse position: direct application of the anterior blade

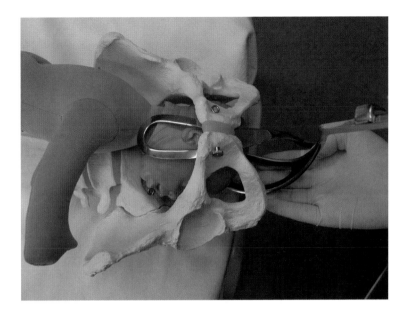

Figure 6.5 Transverse position: direct application of the posterior blade. Once inserted, the blades are locked and asynclitism corrected.

anterior blade is positioned, the posterior blade is passed into the sacral hollow (Figure 6.5). The forceps blade should be slid in close to the head to prevent soft tissue injury. If there is difficulty in applying the posterior blade, often said to be due to the protrusion of the sacral promontory, the blade may be wandered slightly to the side, in front of the sacroiliac joint, then wandered back into the midline. The blades are approximated, asynclitism is corrected and rotation may be then attempted between contractions.

■ **Wandering application.** Where there is difficulty in applying the anterior blade, the anterior blade is first inserted posteriorly, and then wandered over the sinciput or the occiput (classically the sinciput). Once in position, the posterior blade is inserted. Again, asynclitism is corrected before attempting rotation.

Occipito-posterior position

Where the fetal position is OP, the forceps blades are applied directly, in a similar way to that used for traction forceps. The left blade is inserted first after assembling the forceps in front of the perineum and using the direction indicators on the forceps to have them facing the correct way. On applying the right blade, the forceps are approximated and asynclitism corrected. Do not force the forceps in, and do not try to close the forceps against resistance.

Rotation

The first rule for rotation with Kielland's forceps is that it should not be forced. The second rule for rotation with Kielland's forceps is that it should not be forced. That rule is so important that it has been mentioned twice! Rotation takes place usually after slight upwards displacement to disengage the head from the surrounding structures, and then rotation, which is conducted by 'feeling' the way around the pelvis, usually by the shortest route to obtain an anterior position. The essence is that force is not applied – a gentle 'feel' so the head follows the line of least resistance is what is required. Once the head reaches the OA position, a characteristic 'clunk' is often felt through the forceps as the head fits into the pelvis.

Traction

Traction on Kielland's forceps is in the direction of the birth canal. Because of the lack of a pelvic curve on the instrument, this means that traction will be more acutely angled towards the floor. Once the head has descended, traction must follow the angle of the canal around the symphysis pubis, and traction then will be more conventional, almost directly towards the operator, then slightly upwards as the head is delivered over the perineum.

As for the need for an episiotomy, this should be judged individually. Although not routine, one will be required on most occasions.

Complications and how to avoid them

Any OVB will occasionally result in complication. Most are minor. To avoid any serious problems it is important to follow the rules closely and not to deviate from them. Do not force the blades in. Do not try to approximate the blades if they do not fit together properly. Do not force a rotation. Do not squeeze the handles together during traction. Traction should be assessed against descent, but as always, do not pull too hard for too long. Always consider the fetal condition, and do not be afraid to abandon the procedure and perform a caesarean section. Perineal trauma may occur with the use of any forceps, and Kielland's are also reputed to be associated with 'spiral tears' of the vagina. Nerve injuries in the mother are possible but are usually transient. Fetal injury is also uncommon as long as the rules are followed.

Acknowledgements

Thanks to South Warwickshire NHS Trust for the use of the training pelvis.

Photographs by Olivia Oláh.

References

1. Oláh KS. In praise of Kielland's forceps. *BJOG* 2002;109:492–4.

2. Kielland C. The application of forceps to the unrotated head. A description of a new type of forceps and a new method of insertion (translation). *Monatsschrift für Geburtshilfe und Gynäkologie* 1916;43:48–78.

3. Baker PN, Johnson IR. A study of the effect of rotational forceps delivery on fetal acid-base balance. *Acta Obstet Gynecol Scand* 1994;73:787–9.

4. Caughey AB, Sandberg PL, Zlatnik MG, Thiet MP, Parer JT, Laros RK Jr. Forceps compared with vacuum: rates of neonatal and maternal morbidity. *Obstet Gynecol* 2005;106:908–12.

5. Johanson RB, Heycock E, Carter J, Sultan AH, Walklate K, Jones PW. Maternal and child health after assisted vaginal delivery: five-year follow up of a randomised controlled study comparing forceps and ventouse. *BJOG* 1999;106:544–9.

6. Healy DL, Quinn MA, Pepperell RJ. Rotational delivery of the fetus: Kielland's forceps and two other methods compared. *BJOG* 1982;89:501–6.

7. Johanson RB, Menon BKV. Vacuum extraction vs forceps delivery. *Cochrane Database Syst Rev* 2000;(2):CD000224.

8. Johanson RB, Rice C, Doyle M, Arthur J, Anyanwu L, Ibrahim J, et al. A randomised prospective study comparing the new vacuum extractor policy with forceps delivery. *BJOG* 1993;100:524–30.

9. Herabutya Y, O-Prasertsawat P, Boonrangsimant P. Kielland's forceps or ventouse: a comparison. *BJOG* 1988;95:483–7.

10. Chenoy R, Johanson RB. A randomised prospective study comparing delivery with metal and silicone rubber vacuum extractor cups. *BJOG* 1992;96:360–4.

11. Burke N, Field K, Mujahid F, Morrison JJ. Use and safety of Kielland's forceps in current obstetric practice, *Obstet Gynecol*, 2012;120:766–70.

12. Sinha P, Dutta A, Langford K. Instrumental delivery: how to meet the need for improvements in training. *The Obstetrician & Gynaecologist*. 2010;12:265–71.

13. Unterscheider J, McMenamin M, Cullinane F. Rising rates of caesarean deliveries at full cervical dilatation: a concerning trend. *Eur J Obstet Gynecol Reprod Biol* 2011;157:141–4.

14. Oláh KS. Reversal of the decision for caesarean section in the second stage of labour on the basis of consultant vaginal assessment. *J Obstet Gynaecol* 2005;25:115–16.

15. Lewis EA, Barr C, Thomas K. The mode of delivery in women taken to theatre at full dilatation: Does consultant presence make a difference? *J Obstet Gynaecol* 2011;31(3):229–31.

16. *Munro Kerr's Operative Obstetrics, 10th edition.* London: Bailliere Tindall; 1982.

17. Royal College of Obstetricians and Gynaecologists. *Operative vaginal delivery.* Green-top Guideline No. 26. London: RCOG; 2011.

18. Parry-Jones JE. *Kielland's forceps*, London: Butterworth & Co; 1952.

Chapter 7
Caesarean section at full dilatation

Patrick O'Brien and Sadia Bhatti

Key learning points

- To learn about the possible maternal and fetal complications associated with the second-stage caesarean sections.
- Techniques to perform safer second-stage caesarean sections.
- Techniques to identify and deal with the fetal and maternal complications
- Preventative measures that can be adopted to reduce and prevent fetal and maternal complications.

Incidence and epidemiology

There are currently no precise figures for the incidence of caesarean section at full dilatation, but given that there are around 200 000 caesarean births in the UK each year with around 10% at full dilatation, it potentially affects around 20 000 births per year.[1]

According to the audit figures of the RCOG, around 35% of caesareans for singleton pregnancies are performed because of failure to progress in labour, of which one-quarter occur at full cervical dilatation. In 55% of these cases, no attempt was made to achieve a vaginal birth with either forceps or ventouse. In those births where OVB was attempted, the audit found a failure rate of 35% for ventouse and 2% for forceps.[2]

Background

Loudon et al.[3] demonstrated that over the decade from 1992 to 2001, the use of forceps declined whilst the use of the ventouse increased, although this was associated with a higher failure rate. There was an increase in caesarean sections at full dilatation due to both failure of OVB and an increased reluctance to perform it. Whether this is directly attributable to reduced junior doctor hours and, therefore, clinical training and experience, or whether it is simply the continuation of a trend towards lower thresholds for caesarean section, is impossible to decipher. It is noteworthy that, in the 2009 Postgraduate Medical Education and Training Board (PMETB) trainees' survey,[4] 8.8% of trainees said that, if faced with a woman at full dilatation with a fetal malposition and station below the ischial spines, they would expedite birth by caesarean section without an attempt at OVB. This survey showed that an increasing number of women were being taken to theatre at full dilatation, and that in itself may have influenced the mode of birth by lowering the threshold for caesarean section.

Factors that may predispose to caesarean section at full dilatation

Cephalopelvic disproportion

Obstructed labour, the direct clinical consequence of cephalopelvic disproportion (CPD), is responsible for 8% of maternal deaths worldwide, according to figures quoted in the 2005 World Health Report of the World Health Organization (WHO).[5] The report estimates that, in 2000, obstructed labour complicated 4.6% of live births (a total of six million births), resulting in 42 000 maternal deaths, most in sub-Saharan Africa.

Cephalopelvic disproportion (CPD) occurs in a pregnancy where there is a mismatch in size between the fetal head and the maternal pelvis, resulting in failure of the fetus to pass safely through the birth canal for mechanical reasons. This may be caused by the fetal head outgrowing the capacity of the maternal birth canal, or by presentation in a position or attitude that will not allow descent through the pelvis. Untreated, the consequence is obstructed labour, which can endanger the lives of both mother and fetus.

Maternal factors that predispose to CPD include contracted pelvis, pelvic exostoses and spondylolisthesis. Predisposing fetal factors include hydrocephalus, large infant, brow presentation, face presentation (mento-posterior), occipito-posterior (OP) position and deflexed head.

Fetal compromise

The efficacy of electronic fetal monitoring combined with fetal blood gas analysis during labour in identifying fetal compromise was investigated in a retrospective study. OVB for 'fetal distress' diagnosed during labour was performed in 9% of 2659 births. All had continuous electronic fetal heart rate monitoring (EFM) and 22% had a fetal blood analysis. OVB had been performed in 53% of the infants who were acidotic at birth (umbilical artery pH <7.20) and in 46% of those with a low modified Apgar score (<7). These results show that the use of EFM and fetal blood sampling detects fetal compromise without resulting in a high rate of OVB.[6] However, there has been evidence that EFM does increase the likelihood of interventions and one of them could be caesarean section.

High maternal body mass index

Recent studies have shown increase risk of emergency caesarean section in women with a high body mass index (BMI).[7] A meta-analysis of 33 cohort studies showed that the odds ratio (OR) for caesarean section (either elective or emergency) was 1.46 (95% confidence interval [CI] 1.34–1.60) and 2.05 (95% CI 1.86–2.27) among women defined as overweight and obese, respectively, compared with women with a normal weight.[7,8]

Early labour immobilisation/epidural

It has been postulated that epidural anaesthesia may increase the risk of emergency caesarean section, particularly caesarean section at full dilatation, because of impaired ability to push in the second stage. A recent Cochrane systematic review including 21 randomised controlled trials ($n = 6664$ women) compared epidural (all forms) versus nonepidural or no analgesia, and found that the second stage of labour was significantly longer for women with epidural analgesia (ten trials). In addition the incidence of OVB was higher for this group compared with women with nonepidural analgesia or no analgesia. Epidural analgesia was also found to be associated with an increased incidence of oxytocin augmentation, maternal hypotension, maternal fever over 38 °C and urinary retention. However, there was no significant difference in the caesarean section rate between the epidural and nonepidural groups.[9]

Preparation

Appropriate place

An operating theatre with good lighting is a basic prerequisite. Ensure good aseptic technique (because of the increased risk of infection associated with caesarean section at full dilatation) and adequate (preferably experienced) assistance and scrub staff. The most senior obstetrician available should be present, in case of a difficult procedure or repair. An experienced midwife or doctor should be in theatre in case vaginal disimpaction of the fetal head is required.

Analgesia

Before the procedure, discuss with the anaesthetist the likelihood of a difficult procedure. The anaesthetist should be prepared to administer medication to induce uterine relaxation; or to adjust the height or inclination of the operating table, if required. Request in advance that, as well as the oxytocin bolus, an oxytocin infusion should be started as soon as the baby is born.

Consent and WHO checklist

On the consent form, as well as the usual risks of infection, haemorrhage and thrombosis, also document the increased risk of blood transfusion associated with full dilatation caesarean section. During the WHO checklist procedure, ensure that the theatre staff are aware that this is a CS at full dilatation and also of the grade of urgency. Give clear advice about the possible complications, including a potentially difficult birth and haemorrhage.

Examination in the theatre

When the caesarean section is not preceded by a failed OVB, abdominal and vaginal examination before proceeding to caesarean is mandatory as the findings can change quickly in the second stage of labour. This will not cause any significant delay, as it can be performed at the time of insertion of the urinary catheter.

Disimpaction of the fetal head

Before making the skin incision, ensure that an experienced member of staff (midwife or doctor) is allocated to flex and push the head up vaginally, if required. Check that this person is ready and explain to the theatre runners that they may need to help this person access the vagina (by lifting the sterile drapes and flexing the woman's legs). Consider having a fetal pillow available in theatre to aid disimpaction of the fetal head.[10]

Ensure that the neonatologist is aware of the type of caesarean section. (S)he should be present in theatre for the birth, as in second-stage caesarean section there is often an element of fetal compromise and always the possibility of a difficult birth.

Prophylactic antibiotics

Prophylactic intravenous antibiotics should be given for all caesarean sections in line with the National Institute for Health and Care Excellence (NICE) guidelines.[9] As the risk of infection is increased in second-stage compared with first-stage or elective caesarean section, this is of utmost importance. The antibiotic should be given prior to the skin incision as this reduces the risk of infection by 48% compared with giving the antibiotics after clamping of the umbilical cord.[11]

Surgical technique

Uterine incision

The Pfannenstiel incision was introduced in 1900 and is widely used for caesarean section. It has excellent cosmetic results and a low incidence of wound breakdown and allows for early ambulation. The initial cut is made cleanly through the skin, just within the pubic hairline and slightly convex towards the pubis. The fat is incised down to the rectus sheath and the aponeurosis of the external oblique muscle. Short incisions are made on the rectus sheath on either side of the midline and then extended for the full length using scissors. The upper and lower edges of the incision are then grasped in turn and the underlying muscle is separated from the rectus sheath by both blunt and sharp dissection. Caution must be taken to avoid injury to the ilioinguinal and iliohypogastric nerves when extending into the external and internal oblique muscles.

The Joel-Cohen incision is a straight transverse incision, positioned slightly higher than the Pfannenstiel. The subcutaneous tissue is not sharply divided. The anterior rectus sheath is incised in the midline for 3 cm, but the muscles are not separated from the sheath. The peritoneum is bluntly opened in a transverse direction.

The Pfannenstiel and Joel-Cohen techniques were compared.[12] Less fever, pain, blood loss, analgesic requirements and postoperative morbidity, as well as shorter operating time, were demonstrated in the Joel-Cohen incision group.

Bladder reflection

As there is an increased risk of extension of the uterine incision during birth, the bladder should be reflected well down, both centrally and laterally (most extensions are at the lateral angles of the incision).

Identification of lower uterine segment

Care must be taken to identify correctly the true level of the lower uterine segment. Use the uterovesical reflection of the visceral peritoneum as a landmark, as the bladder may be higher than expected when the cervix is fully dilated.

Opening the uterine cavity

After reflecting the bladder well down, make a careful uterine incision. Make this incision a little higher than usual (but still in the lower segment) so as to ensure that you are clear of the fully dilated cervix and vagina. The lower segment is likely to be thin, so incise carefully so as not to cut the baby. Having made a superficial incision, attempt to enter the uterus using a finger rather than the knife. Keep the initial incision small; there may be some benefit in making it U-shaped. If the lower segment is very thin, consider extending the initial incision laterally with a pair of scissors in a U-shape. This creates an adequate opening for birth while reducing the chances of an uncontrolled tear caused by stretching the incision manually. It also helps to direct the incision (and any tear) away from the uterine arteries, which ascend the lateral aspect of the uterus.

As you make the uterine incision be aware that, as the fetal head is low in the pelvis, the fetal arm may present. Be prepared to prevent the arm from delivering first. If this does occur, the arm should be replaced into the uterus (and held there) before attempting to deliver the head.

Previous abdominal surgery

In women who have had previous abdominal surgery, anticipate that entry and bladder reflection may be more difficult and ensure that senior help is available. When the bladder is adherent, take time (assuming there is no urgency) to ensure adequate bladder dissection and reflection. If the bladder is not adequately reflected before birth, and there is a significant extension of the uterine incision, complications may occur. Firstly, the adherent bladder may tear along with the uterus. Secondly, even if the bladder is not damaged, it may be necessary to dissect it off of the torn lower segment to gain access to the uterine tear. This dissection will be far more difficult to perform than if it had been done prior to birth.

Delivery of the fetal head

Follow these steps:

1. Introduce a hand below the baby's head.
2. Flex the baby's head. If the position is occipito-anterior (OA), this is usually simple. If the position is OP, a common cause of obstructed labour, this may be more difficult. Make sure that you introduce your hand around the baby's head until you can feel the occiput; only then should you try to flex it.
3. Disimpact the head (see below).
4. Deliver the head through the uterine incision.

Do not skip any of these four steps: missing a step will make the birth more difficult and extension of the uterine incision more likely. For example, if you try to disimpact an OP head before flexing it, it may result in further deflexion but no disimpaction. If you try to deliver the baby's head before disimpacting, it will lead to extension of the uterine incision.

The height of the operating table

The aim is to have the table low enough that you can keep your arm straight during delivery of the head. If the head is very impacted, this makes manipulation and disimpaction easier.

Disimpacting the fetal head

Your hand should be below the fetal head at the occiput. Attempt to disimpact only after you have successfully flexed the head, particularly when it is in an OP position. Apply traction in the maternal long axis, i.e. towards the mother's head. Do not attempt to deliver the baby's head at this stage. A 'suction' sound is often heard as the pressure seal is broken (Figure 7.1).

Measures to be taken if there is difficulty in disimpacting the fetal head

At this stage, if the surgeon has difficulty in disimpacting the baby's head from above, the assistant (who should be standing by) can be asked to flex and push up the baby's head vaginally. This pressure should be spread over as many fingers as possible, in order to minimise the risk of trauma to the fetal skull. Ideally, this person should introduce his or her whole hand into the vagina. In addition, if necessary, the scrubbed assistant can help by applying pressure on the fetal shoulders (again pushing towards the mother's head), which are often at the level of the uterine incision in this situation.

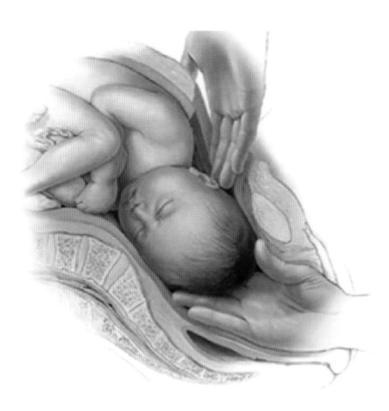

Figure 7.1 Disimpacting the fetal head. Disimpaction should be attempted only after the head has been successfully flexed, particularly when it is in an occiput posterior position

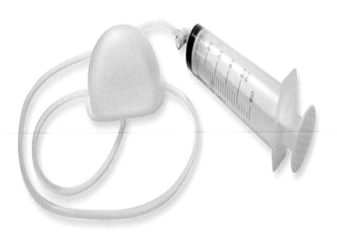

Figure 7.2 The fetal pillow is inflated with water and can help with the head disimpaction

A uterine relaxant can be administered by the anaesthetist, according to local guidelines.

Use of a 'fetal pillow' may help in this situation (Figure 7.2). This consists of a balloon that can be introduced into the vagina and inflated with water,

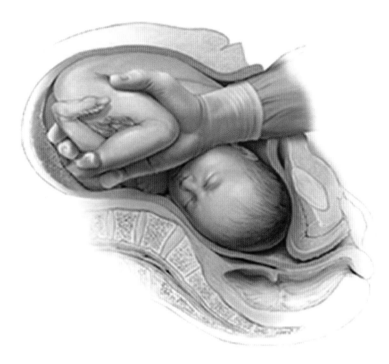

Figure 7.3 If disimpacting the head proves impossible, an alternative is to grasp a leg and deliver the fetus as breech

thereby pushing up on the impacted head. The potential advantage, compared with pushing up by hand, is that the pressure is gradual and the force spread more evenly over the baby's head. The aim is to disimpact the head, allowing easier delivery at caesarean section. It may also reduce the risk of skull fracture as the balloon spreads the force more equally, although further evidence is needed to support these suggested benefits.[11]

Reverse breech birth

Delivering the fetus as a breech is an alternative when disimpacting the head proves impossible (Figure 7.3). Schwake et al.[13] showed that this technique is feasible and carries a low risk of maternal and neonatal morbidity. Previous studies examining the reverse breech manoeuvre during second-stage caesarean section have found this method preferable to the abdominovaginal approach or the push method.[14,15] Inadvertent extension of the uterine incision and maternal postpartum complications were more prevalent in the push method than the reverse breech approach.

Maternal complications

Extension of the uterine angles

In this situation, exteriorising the uterus is helpful. It allows better visualisation of the angles and any tears, and makes access for the repair much easier.

By placing the uterine arteries under tension, it also reduces the amount of bleeding. Always advise the anaesthetist in advance when you need to exteriorise the uterus, as it may make the woman uncomfortable and may cause some vagal stimulation, leading to the woman feeling faint or nauseous.

- A second assistant is valuable to help provide better exposure when there are suspected extensions.
- If required, call for help of adequate seniority early.
- Identify the apex at each end of the uterine incision.
- Ensure that the bladder is reflected well down, i.e. clear of the uterine incision and any tears.
- Identify the ureters, particularly when the tear extends inferolaterally (which is common).

If there is significant bleeding and difficult access, it is preferable to begin the repair with a blunt Vicryl™ number 1 suture, as it reduces the chances of a needle-stick injury to the surgeon or (more commonly) the assistant. However, when the tissues are very friable, a sharp needle may be more appropriate for precise placement of sutures.

Occasionally, when the apex of a tear descends deep into the pelvis and cannot be reached, the first suture should be placed as low as possible in the tear, leaving the tied end of the suture long. Once tied, the two ends of the suture can then be used to pull upwards on the tear; then another suture can be placed lower down. In this way, the suture can be advanced step-wise until the apex of the tear is reached.

Extension into the broad ligament

The possibility of extension into the broad ligament should always be borne in mind and checked for. The accumulation of blood may not initially be obvious. If on palpation there is suspicion of a broad ligament haematoma, the broad ligament should be opened. Pressure and Vicryl 2/0 can be used to achieve haemostasis.

Cervical or high vaginal lacerations

An extension of the uterine incision may be directed downwards and involve the cervix (which is fully dilated so often close to the uterine incision) and even vagina (which at full dilatation is continuous with the lower segment). In this situation, it sometimes proves impossible to achieve complete repair from above (abdominally). In this case, the woman may need a combined abdominal and vaginal repair in the lithotomy position with two experienced operators, one at the abdominal incision and other operating vaginally. There is a significant risk of ureteric (or even urethral) involvement; if this occurs, the urology team should be involved.

Damage to bladder or ureter

Damage to the bladder or ureter is more likely in situations of downwards extension of a uterine tear, either laterally or anteriorly. Accidental involvement of a ureter in a suture is more likely when the anatomy is distorted by the tear, particularly when there is poor visualisation of the operative field due to bleeding or because it is deep in the pelvis. Exteriorisation of the uterus will help to avoid such trauma. Careful identification of the ureters and bladder is essential, and there should always be a high index of suspicion in such situations. If any damage to the bladder or ureters is detected (or suspected), a urological opinion should be sought. Methylene blue dye can be injected into the bladder via the urinary catheter to identify any leakage. This dye should be available in all obstetric theatres.

Postpartum haemorrhage and blood transfusion

Postpartum haemorrhage and blood transfusion are more common because of an increased likelihood of uterine atony and trauma.[16]

Further surgery

Further surgery is more common (eg. bladder repair and hysterectomy) as well as repair of genital tract tears and extensions.[16]

Sepsis

Sepsis is more common following emergency than elective caesarean section, particularly following caesarean section at full dilatation.[16] Prophylactic antibiotics, which should be given prior to the uterine incision, reduce this risk.[11]

VTE

VTE is a leading cause of maternal mortality. Prophylaxis should be prescribed following second stage CS.

Admission to intensive care unit

Admission to intensive care unit (ICU) is more common because of the complications mentioned above, in particular haemorrhage and sepsis.[16]

Fetal complications

Skull fracture

Skull fracture may occasionally occur during difficult disimpaction of the fetal head during a second-stage caesarean section.

Fetal limb fractures

Limb fracture is uncommon during birth of a term baby but more likely in a difficult preterm birth. Studies have shown that there is no increase in the incidence of fractures in reverse breech deliveries during caesarean section.[14,15]

Advanced resuscitation

Compared with caesarean birth at less than full dilatation, babiés born by CS at full dilatation were 1.5 times more likely to require advanced resuscitation. However, no differences were seen in the rates of neonatal trauma, low 5-minute Apgar score or neonatal sepsis.[17]

Prevention of complications of second-stage caesarean section

Training

Desperate Debra® (simulated training)[18]

The Desperate Debra® model (Figure 7.4) simulates the abdomen, uterus and fetus of a birthing mother, and has a mechanism to replicate an impacted fetal head.

Education and training towards gaining the following skills are possible:

- successful delivery of an impacted fetal head at caesarean section (with adjustable degrees of difficulty)
- vaginal examination in advanced labour
- identification of fetal head position and variable degrees of flexion and asynclitism – the model has palpable fontanelles and sutures.

Interactive courses

Labour ward supervision and early senior involvement

Labour ward supervision and early senior involvement to improve rotational OVB will help reduce the incidence of full dilatation caesarean section.

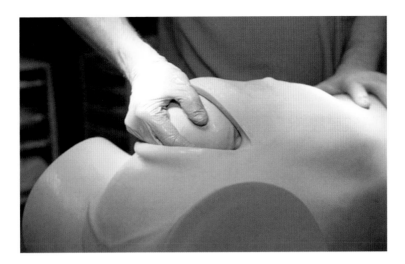

Figure 7.4 The Desperate Debra® model allows the simulation of disimpacting and delivering the fetal head. Photograph courtesy of Adam Rouilly.

Debriefing

Good communication with the parents throughout the birth is essential. When the obstetrician is preoccupied, the supporting midwife or anaesthetist should take on this role. After the birth, preferably the same day or the following day at the latest, it is good practice for the most senior obstetrician involved to debrief the couple about the events around birth. Second-stage caesarean sections can be associated with a series of events occurring in rapid succession and the parents can be left confused about exactly what happened and why. It is important that the clinicians involved take the time to explain the events clearly to the parents so they fully understand what happened and the reasons for any difficulties. The possibility of vaginal birth for subsequent pregnancies should also be discussed at this stage.

Documentation

It is responsibility of the operating surgeon and anaesthetist to ensure that all relevant documentation is completed. This will include the operating notes, an adverse incident reporting form, and any relevant proformas in use in the unit. Ensure that correct timings of events are recorded; it is valuable to designate a scribe whose role is to document events and timings in real time during the procedure. Where indicated, illustrative diagrams of any extensive tears and repairs should be included, as these may be helpful in the management of future pregnancies.

Points to remember

Table 7.1 Points to remember

Preoperatively	Be prepared	Get appropriate help
Intraoperatively	Stay calm	Do not fight the uterine cavity
	Communicate with your anaesthetist	Compression: pressure on bleeders not the suction
	Reflect bladder well down before uterine incision	Uterine incision a little higher than usual
	Consider extending uterine incision with scissors	Watch for, and prevent, delivery of a presenting arm when opening the uterus
	Always flex the head well before attempting to disimpact	Always disimpact the head completely from the pelvis before attempting to deliver the baby
	Exteriorise the uterus if there is a significant tear or heavy bleeding	Get urological support if there is suspicion of damage to the urinary tract
Postoperatively	Be prepared for postpartum haemorrhage	
	Sepsis	Antibiotics as required
	Check for perineal trauma, if appropriate (e.g. failed operative vaginal birth)	

References

1. UK Statistics for Caesarean Sections from the Office for National Statistics, *Births in England and Wales* 2009 [www.statistics.gov.uk/statbase and www.isdscot.org].

2. Royal College of Obstetricians and Gynaecolgists Clinical Effectiveness Support Unit. *The National Sentinel Caesarean Section Audit Report*. London: RCOG Press; 2001.

3. Loudon JA, Groom KM, Hinkson L, Harrington D, Paterson-Brown S. Changing trends in operative delivery performed at full dilatation over a 10-year period. *J Obstet Gynaecol* 2010;30:370–5.

4. PMETB 2008–2009 Trainees Survey [www.gmc-uk.org/ National_Training_Surveys_2008_09_20090929.pdf_30512348.pdf].

5. Make every mother and child count, *The World Health Report* 2005 [whqlibdoc.who.int/whr/ 2005/9241562900].

6. van den berg P, Schimdt S, Gesche J, Saling E. Fetal distress and the condition of the newborn using cardiotocography and fetal blood analysis. *Br J Obstet Gynaecol* 1987;94:72–5.

7. Centre for Maternal and Child Enquiries, Royal College of Obstetricians and Gynaecologists. *Management of Women with Obesity in Pregnancy. CMACE/RCOG Joint Guideline*. London: CMACE, RCOG; 2010.

8. Zhang J, Bricker L, Wray S, Quenby S. Poor uterine contractility in obese women. *BJOG* 2007;114:343–8.

9. National Institute for Health and Care Excellence. Intrapartum care: *Care of healthy women and their babies during childbirth*. London:NICE; 2007.

10. Verma R, Mandeep S. New developments, reducing complications of a deeply engaged head at second stage caesarean. A simple instrument. *The Obstetrician & Gynaecologist*, 2008;10:38–41.

11. Kittur ND, McMullen KM, Russo AJ, Ruhl L, Kay HH, Warren DK. Long-term effect of infection prevention practices and case mix on cesarean surgical site infections. *Obstet Gynecol* 2012;120:246–51.

12. Karanth KL, Sathish N. Review of advantages of Joel-Cohen surgical abdominal incision in caesarean section: a basic science perspective. *Med J Malaysia* 2010;65:204–8.

13. Schwake D, Petchenkin L, Younis JS. Reverse breech extraction in cases of second stage caesarean section. *J Obstet Gynaecol* 2012;32:548–51.

14. Fasubaa OB, Ezechi OC, Orji EO, Ogunniyi SO, Akindele ST, Loto OM, et al. Delivery of the impacted head of the fetus at caesarean section after prolonged obstructed labour: a randomized comparative study of two methods. *J Obstet Gynaecol* 2002;22:375–8.

15. Chopra S, Bagga R, Keepanasseril A, Jain V, Kalra J, Suri V. Disengagement of the deeply engaged fetal head during cesarean section in advanced labor: conventional method versus reverse breech extraction. *Acta Obstet Gynecol Scand* 2009;88:1163–6.

16. McKelvey A, Ashe R, McKenna D, Roberts R. Caesarean section in the second stage of labour: a retrospective review of obstetric setting and morbidity. *J Obstet Gynaecol* 2010;30:264–7.

17. Allen VM, O'Connell CM, Baskett TF. Maternal and perinatal morbidity of caesarean delivery at full cervical dilatation compared with caesarean delivery in the first stage of labour. *BJOG* 2005;112:986–90.

18. *Desperate Debra® – Impacted Fetal Head Simulator* (www.adam-rouilly.co.uk/productdetails).

Chapter 8
Medico-legal matters

Fraser McLeod and Tim Draycott

Key learning points

■ To explore the potential medico-legal implications of operative vaginal birth (OVB).

■ To outline strategies to reduce risk to both mother and infant through safe OVB.

Operative vaginal birth (OVB) is considered to be one of the six critical functions of basic emergency obstetric care according to the World Health Organization (WHO) and the United Nations.[1] Despite these recommendations, OVB rates have declined over the last 30 years in many developed and developing world settings.[2,3]

There has been a problem with perceived safety of OVB and the US Food and Drug Administration (FDA), which issued a health advisory reporting neonatal injuries/deaths following vacuum birth, highlighted this in 1998. However, more recent data have confirmed that when women get to the second stage of labour, and birth needs to be expedited, a single-instrument application is the safest method of birth, followed by a caesarean section, then two instrument applications (ventouse and forceps), with failed OVB leading to caesarean section being the least safe.[4]

There is a balance of risks and benefits with operative birth; obstetricians are often faced with the dilemma of making a difficult choice between OVB and caesarean section when birth needs to be expedited at full cervical dilatation. Operative vaginal birth is associated with similar rates of serious neonatal complications compared with caesarean birth at full dilatation;[5] however, OVB can often be expedited more quickly.[6] Even for experienced clinicians, this decision-making process can be extremely challenging, and this is particularly the case where experience with operative birth is limited.

There is now clear guidance from the RCOG and other colleges for both decision making about, and performance of, operative birth, and these have become the standard of care.

Potential areas for litigation

Litigation is often complex and the use of instruments alone is seldom the only factor in a medico-legal action; however, the following are some of the more common claims against obstetricians after completed or attempted OVB:

■ inappropriate indication and/or conditions for safe OVB

■ inappropriate instrument

■ incorrect technique and application of instruments

■ procedure failure

■ failure to anticipate impending complications

■ maternal complications

■ fetal complications

■ inadequate consent and poor communication.

In the following section, we discuss these potential litigation areas in detail and outline strategies that clinicians can adopt to optimise safe clinical practice and improve outcomes for mothers and their babies.

How to minimise adverse outcomes

Reduce the rate of operative vaginal birth

Ideally, OVB should be avoided, particularly where better care in labour can improve the likelihood of a spontaneous vaginal birth.

There are a number of strategies that have been identified to reduce the requirement for intervention and the RCOG Green-top Guideline for 'Operative vaginal delivery' recommends the following:

■ All women should be encouraged to have continuous support during labour.

■ Use of a partogram, use of upright or lateral positions and avoiding epidural analgesia will reduce the need for operative vaginal delivery.

■ Oxytocin in primiparous women with epidurals will decrease the need for operative vaginal delivery.

■ Delayed pushing in primiparous women with an epidural will reduce the risk of rotational and midcavity deliveries.[7]

Ensure that operative intervention is indicated

Operative intervention is employed to expedite birth, for fetal and/or maternal indications and where the benefits of OVB significantly outweigh the risks of operative intervention and/or continued pushing.

These indications are identified and summarised in Table 8.1, taken from the RCOG's Green-top Guideline on 'Operative vaginal delivery'.[7]

The two most common indications, presumed fetal compromise and inadequate progress in labour, have been defined in the National Institute for Health and Care Excellence (NICE) intrapartum care guideline[8] and they are recapped below.

Table 8.1 Indications for operative vaginal delivery

Type	Indication
Fetal	Presumed fetal compromise
Maternal	To shorten and reduce the effects of the second stage of labour on medical conditions (e.g. cardiac disease class III or IV*, hypertensive crises, myasthenia gravis, spinal cord injury, patients at risk of autonomic dysreflexia, proliferative retinopathy)
Inadequate progress	Nulliparous women – lack of continuing progress for 3 hours (total of active and passive second-stage labour) with regional anaesthesia, or 2 hours without regional anaesthesia
	Multiparous women – lack of continuing progress for 2 hours (total of active and passive second-stage labour) with regional anaesthesia, or 1 hour without regional anaesthesia
	Maternal fatigue/exhaustion

* New York Heart Association classification. No indication is absolute and each case should be considered individually. Reproduced with permission from the RCOG Green-top Guideline on 'Operative vaginal delivery'.

Fetal compromise

A complete review of electronic fetal monitoring (EFM) is beyond the scope of this chapter, and indeed book; however, a sticker is included for cardiotocography (CTG) interpretation that is consistent with the NICE intrapartum guideline, published in 2007, Figure 8.1.[8]

The management of a pathological CTG is clearly defined in the NICE intrapartum guideline[8] and in most circumstances it would be appropriate to expedite birth in the second stage rather than perform fetal blood sampling, when the CTG is pathological.

Delay in the second stage of labour

Expected minimum progress in the second stage of labour is also clearly defined by the NICE intrapartum guideline,[8] as is a proposed model for the timing of intervention. Delay in the second stage of labour varies with parity.

- Nulliparous women:
  - ☐ Birth would be expected to take place within 3 hours of the start of the active second stage in most women.
  - ☐ A diagnosis of delay in the active second stage should be made when it has lasted 2 hours and women should be referred to a healthcare professional trained to undertake an OVB if birth is not imminent.
- Parous women:
  - ☐ Birth would be expected to take place within 2 hours of the start of the active second stage in most women.
  - ☐ A diagnosis of delay in the active second stage should be made when it has lasted 1 hour and women should be referred to a healthcare professional trained to undertake an OVB if birth is not imminent (recommendation 1.7.3).

Therefore, the NICE intrapartum guideline should be used as the standard of care for both of the most common indications for OVB; fetal compromise and delay in the second stage of labour.

Ensure operative vaginal birth is the safest option

Caesarean section is a reasonable option in the second stage of labour when OVB is deemed inappropriate or unsafe. However, caesarean section also carries significant, and sometimes preventable, morbidity for the mother and her baby.

113

Intrapartum CTG Proforma	Reassuring (Acceptable)	Non-reassuring	Abnormal	
Baseline rate (bpm)	110 – 160 Rate:	100 – 109 Rate: 161 – 180 Rate:	Less than 100 Rate: More than 180 Rate: Sinusoidal pattern for 10 minutes or more	Comments:-
N.B Rising baseline rate even within normal range may be of concern if other non-reassuring / abnormal features present.				
Variability (bpm)	5 bpm or more	Less than 5 bpm for 40 - 90 minutes	Less than 5 bpm for 90 minutes	Comments:-
Accelerations	Present	None for 40 mins	Comments	
Decelerations	None	Typical variable decelerations with more than 50% of contractions for more than 90 minutes	Atypical variable decelerations with more than 50% of contractions for more than 30 minutes	Comments:-
	Typical variable decelerations with more than 50% of contractions but for less than 90 minutes	Atypical variable decelerations with more than 50% of contractions for less than 30 minutes	Late decelerations for more than 30 minutes	
	Typical or atypical variable decelerations with less than 50% of contractions	Late decelerations for less than 30 minutes		
	True early decelerations	Single prolonged deceleration for up to 3 minutes	Single prolonged deceleration for more than 3 minutes	

N.B If CTG has any non-reassuring or abnormal features present from commencement of monitoring, it may not be appropriate to wait 30 or 90 minutes before requesting review

Opinion	*Normal CTG* (All 4 features reassuring)	*Suspicious CTG* (1 non-reassuring feature)	*Pathological CTG* (2 or more non-reassuring or 1 or more abnormal features)	
Cont's: :10	Maternal pulse:	Liquor colour:	Dilatation (cm):	Gestation (wks):

Action:

Date: .... Time: .... Signature: .... Print: .... Designation: ....

Figure 8.1 Example of an Intrapartum CTG sticker based on the NICE Intrapartum Care Guidelines

Caesarean section at full dilatation is associated with an increased risk of major obstetric haemorrhage, prolonged hospital stay and neonatal special care baby unit (SCBU) admission compared with completed instrumental birth.[4] Moreover, OVB, when successful, requires reduced analgesia requirement, can be expedited more quickly[6] and women are much more likely (>80%) to have a spontaneous vaginal birth in their next pregnancy.[9,10] In addition, repeat caesarean section may limit maternal choice in future pregnancies and also increases the risk of abnormal placentation, which carries significant maternal risks.[11]

Therefore, OVB may often be the best option for the mother and baby in the second stage of labour, but it is essential that the accoucheur performs a careful, accurate and comprehensive clinical assessment to confirm that the prerequisite conditions are met for safe vaginal operative delivery.

Table 8.2 summaries the RCOG recommended prerequisites for safe OVB.

There are also contraindications to OVB:

- Relative contraindications:
  - ☐ Fetal bleeding disorders (e.g. alloimmune thrombocytopenia)
  - ☐ Predisposition to fracture (e.g. osteogenesis imperfecta)
  - ☐ Blood-borne viral infection of the mother.
- Absolute contraindications:
  - ☐ Face presentation (ventouse only).
  - ☐ Gestation <34 weeks.
  - ☐ Gestation 34–36 weeks (ventouse only).

Trial of operative vaginal birth in theatre

Where difficult OVB is anticipated, particularly where there is a significant risk of failure, a trial of OVB can be undertaken in theatre with immediate recourse to caesarean section, if necessary. A recent study demonstrated that if immediate recourse to caesarean section was available following failed OVB, there was no evidence of increased morbidity risk to the mother or the fetus compared with those who proceeded directly to caesarean section; therefore, it is a reasonable option for selected women.[7]

Higher rates of failure are associated with:

- maternal body mass index (BMI) >30
- estimated fetal weight over 4000 g or clinically big baby

Table 8.2 Prerequisites for operative vaginal delivery (reproduced with permission from the RCOG Green-top Guideline on 'Operative vaginal delivery')

Full abdominal and vaginal examination	Head is less than or equal to one-fifth palpable per abdomen.
	Vertex presentation.
	Cervix is fully dilated and the membranes ruptured.
	Exact position of the head can be determined so proper placement of the instrument can be achieved.
	Assessment of caput and moulding.
	Pelvis is deemed adequate. Irreducible moulding may indicate cephalopelvic disproportion.
Preparation of mother	Clear explanation should be given and informed consent obtained.
	Appropriate analgesia is in place for midcavity rotational deliveries. This will usually be a regional block. A pudendal block may be appropriate, particularly in the context of urgent delivery.
	Maternal bladder has been emptied recently. Indwelling catheter should be removed or balloon deflated.
	Aseptic technique.
Preparation of staff	Operator must have the knowledge, experience and skill necessary.
	Adequate facilities are available (appropriate equipment, bed, lighting).
	Back-up plan in place in case of failure to deliver. When conducting midcavity deliveries, theatre staff should be immediately available to allow a caesarean section to be performed without delay (less than 30 minutes). A senior obstetrician competent in performing midcavity deliveries should be present if a junior trainee is performing the delivery.
	Anticipation of complications that may arise (e.g. shoulder dystocia, postpartum haemorrhage).
	Personnel present who are trained in neonatal resuscitation.

- occipito-posterior (OP) position
- midcavity birth or when one-fifth of the head palpable per abdomen.

Therefore, these can be considered indications to perform the OVB in theatre; however, the threshold for moving to theatre will vary with the confidence and expertise of individual practitioners.

Use the correct instrument

In the 1980s, most OVBs were by forceps (83% forceps deliveries in 1989). However, by 2000, this had decreased to under half. By contrast, the rate of ventouse birth has more than doubled in the last two decades. Some speculate that this reversing trend is likely to be secondary to the operator's concerns regarding instrument-related maternal complications, in particular pelvic floor injuries.

A Cochrane systematic review of nine randomised controlled studies evaluated the merits of vacuum extraction versus forceps birth.[12] Forceps were less likely than the ventouse to fail to achieve a vaginal birth with the allocated instrument (risk ratio 0.65, 95% confidence interval [CI] 0.45–0.94). However, with forceps there was a trend to more caesarean sections, and significantly more third- or fourth-degree tears (with or without episiotomy), vaginal trauma, use of general anaesthesia, and flatus incontinence or altered continence. Facial injury was more likely with forceps (risk ratio 5.10, 95% CI 1.12–23.25). Using a random effects model because of heterogeneity between studies, there was a trend towards fewer cases of cephalhaematoma with forceps (average risk ratio 0.64, 95% CI 0.37–1.11).

Among different types of ventouse, the metal cup was more likely to result in a successful vaginal birth than the soft cup, with more cases of scalp injury and cephalhaematoma. The hand-held ventouse was associated with more failures than the metal ventouse, and a trend to fewer failures than the soft ventouse.

Overall, forceps or the metal cup appear to be most effective at achieving a vaginal birth, but with increased risk of maternal trauma with forceps and neonatal trauma with the metal cup.[13]

It is also important to note that there is a wide variation in the type of forceps and vacuum extraction instruments that are available for use. There are over 700 models of forceps and the choice is often subjective. There are no randomised controlled trials comparing different types of forceps.

Rotational forceps such as Kielland's carry additional risks and their use requires specific training and expertise; however, a recent study has confirmed that the use of Kielland's forceps is associated with a high successful birth rate and apparently low maternal and neonatal morbidity.[14] Therefore, their use is reasonable and appropriate in skilled hands. Alternatively, rotational vacuum extraction or manual rotation, followed by forceps, can be performed.

Rigid vacuum cups are more likely to result in vaginal birth than soft cups, but they are more likely to cause scalp trauma. Therefore, the choice of instrument is dependent on the specifics of the clinical situation and the experience of the accoucheur. Ultimately, the most important determining factor should be the operator's preference based on his/her skill and experience.

Ensure right technique, adequate training and/or supervision

An OVB should be performed by an operator who has the experience and skills necessary to perform an adequate clinical assessment, use the instruments safely and manage complications that may arise.

System analysis of litigation claims often reveals inadequate training as a major contributor to adverse outcomes.[15] Neonatal trauma is increased with initial unsuccessful attempts at OVB by inexperienced operators and improved training of obstetricians for OVB has been recommended.[16]

The RCOG has recommended dedicated consultant sessions on the labour ward, which they suggest should facilitate better training and supervision of trainees and a higher proportion of OVBs being performed by experienced obstetricians. Assessment of clinical competence is an important element of training.

The RCOG has a system of training and competency assessment for all trainees in their training logbook and it would be reasonable to ask for evidence that a trainee has been both appropriately trained and certified to perform the OVB, either alone or under supervision.

Know when to abandon

The RCOG Green-top Guideline for operative vaginal delivery recommends that the attempted OVB should be abandoned where there is no evidence of progressive descent with moderate traction during each contraction or where birth is not imminent following three contractions of a correctly applied instrument by an experienced operator.[7]

The RCOG guideline also explains that the bulk of malpractice litigation results from a failure to abandon the procedure at the appropriate time, particularly the failure to eschew prolonged, repeated or excessive traction with poor progress.

If there is difficulty in applying the instrument correctly, no descent with each traction, birth is not imminent following three pulls and/or a reasonable time has elapsed since the decision for intervention has been made, then the attempt at OVB should be abandoned.

Be careful when considering sequential instruments

The use of multiple instruments is associated with increased neonatal trauma[7] and therefore the use of two instruments should be avoided.

However, the use of outlet/low-cavity forceps following failed vacuum extraction may be appropriate in avoiding potentially complex caesarean section providing delivery is imminent. Indeed, in a recent randomised study of ventouse delivery in a UK unit there was a failure rate of primary ventouse delivery of >27% and forceps were employed after ventouse in 16% of births.[17]

Anticipate severe perineal injuries

The RCOG guideline for third- and fourth-degree tears recognises that they are neither predictable nor preventable.[18]

The Hands On Or Poised (HOOP) study, published in 1998, demonstrated that there were no differences in third- and fourth-degree perineal tears in two groups of women randomised to two different methods of midwifery management of the second stage, including a 'hands off' method.[19]

Episiotomy does not prevent third- and fourth-degree tears after OVB[20] and may increase the rate of third- and fourth-degree tears in normal vaginal birth, particularly midline episiotomies.[18]

Identification

All women should be examined in a systematic manner to identify the extent of any perineal tears as defined in the NICE intrapartum guideline.[8]

The RCOG guideline for repair of third- and fourth-degree perineal tears published in March 2007[18] mandates that all women having an operative vaginal birth or who have experienced perineal injury should be examined by an experienced practitioner trained in the recognition and management of perineal tears.

Andrews et al.[21] has established that 25% of third- and fourth-degree tears could be missed by doctors and the third-degree tear rate doubled when every perineal tear was examined by a second experienced person.[22] If the appropriate examination is performed then third/fourth-degree perineal tears will almost certainly be identified. In a recent series of 250 vaginal births, only one woman had an occult external sphincter injury that was not detectable at the time of birth.[21]

A recent review of 10 years of National Health Service Litigation Authority (NHSLA) claims identified that in regard to claims concerning women, perineal trauma is one of the largest areas of litigation.[15] They concluded that training remains a crucial factor in diagnosing the existence and severity of tears following birth and from a legal perspective, ensuring a thorough examination is performed, including the extent of which is documentation.

The RCOG has a system of training and competency assessment for the identification and management of perineal tears for all trainees in their training logbook and in the event of an injury it would be reasonable to ask for evidence that a trainee had been both appropriately trained and certified. Therefore, severe perineal injury is unpreventable; however, it should be recognised.

Good communication

Poor maternal experience is another significant complication of pregnancy and birth. UK-based research showed that over 25% of new mothers were not satisfied with communication by the medical staff and there was a significant association between satisfaction with communication by medical staff and overall satisfaction with care.[23]

Communication with parents can be improved after training using patient actors[24,25] and it is noteworthy that the patient actors in a study reported that their perception of their safety during the drill could improved by information provided about the:

■ cause of emergency

■ condition of the baby

■ aims of treatment.

The RCOG Guideline for 'Operative Vaginal Delivery'[7] mandates that informed consent must be obtained and clear explanation given. The RCOG provides a patient information sheet for OVB and it may be appropriate to provide a consent form with standardised risks.

The threat of litigation affects the everyday decision-making process of practising clinicians. However, effective communication is one of the most effective risk-management tools. Good communication with the patient as well as other members of the team will aid the clinician to minimise the risk of morbidity and, where morbidity occurs, to minimise the likelihood of litigation, without limiting maternal choice.

Ensure good documentation

Defending a potential claim can be extremely difficult unless there is good documentation for the operative birth, including indications, examination findings and performance of the OVB or CS.

Judges or experts reviewing a case often deem that meticulous documentation reflects meticulous care and also 'If it isn't documented then it didn't happen'. The quality of documentation can reflect a clinician's level of professionalism and forms the basis of any successful defence of a claim or complaint. Claims are twice as likely to be successfully defended if documentation is judged to be adequate.

After-the-fact verbal explanations can have the appearance of an effort to escape consequences.

Good record keeping is also essential for communication, education, clinical audit and risk-management purposes. The following elements of the birth should be documented and a standardised proforma may help:

■ Indication for procedure
■ Consent
■ Preprocedure assessment
  ☐ Abdominal palpation
  ☐ Position and station of the fetal head
  ☐ Degree of caput and moulding
  ☐ Fetal heart assessment
  ☐ Bladder emptied
■ Ease of application of instrument
■ Type of rotation
■ Number of pulls
■ Use of sequential instruments

OPERATIVE VAGINAL DELIVERY RECORD

Patient Details

Date ....

Operator   Name ....   Grade ....

Supervisor   Name ....   Grade ....

Indication(s) for delivery: ....

Classification of OVD: outlet / low / midcavity   **Rotation > 45°:** yes / no

Fetal wellbeing: CTG: normal / suspicious / pathological   **Liquor:** clear / meconium

---

Prerequisites:

Place of delivery: room / theatre

Analgesia: local / pudendal / regional

Consent: verbal / written

Catheterised: yes / no

Examination

1/5th per abdomen: ....

Dilatation:..

Position: ....

Station: ....

Moulding: ....

Caput:..

Procedure

Instrument used:

Vacuum extractor : silastic / Kiwi / metal anterior / metal posterior

Forceps: rotational / non-rotational / outlet

Number of pulls: ....

Traction: easy / moderate / strong

Maternal effort: minimal / moderate / good

Placenta: CCT/ manual

Episiotomy: yes / no

Perineal tear:
- 1st degree ☐
- 2nd degree ☐
- 3rd / 4th degree ☐ (complete pro forma)
- Other ☐ (complete suturing pro forma if necessary)

Multiple instrument use: yes / no
Examination before second instrument
1/5th per abdomen:............................
Position: ....
Station: ....
Moulding: ....
Caput:..
Reasons for second instrument:
....
....
....

EBL: ....

Baby: M / F Birth weight:.......... (kg) Apgar: 1..... 5..... 10.....   **Cord pH:** Arterial.......... Venous..........

Post-delivery care:

Level of care: routine / high dependency

Syntocinon infusion: yes / no

Catheter: yes / no   Remove ....

Vaginal pack: yes / no   Remove ....

Diclofenac 100 mg PR: yes / no Analgesia prescribed: yes / no

Thromboembolic risk: low / medium / high

Thromboprophylaxis prescribed: yes / no

Signature: ....   Date: ....

RCOG Green-top Guideline No. 26   17 of 19   © Royal College of Obstetricians and Gynaecologists

Figure 8.2 Example operative vaginal delivery pro forma

- Condition of the baby
- Assessment of vagina and perineum post birth
- Paired cord pH results.
- Assessment of maternal VTE risk.

The Clinical Negligence Scheme for Trusts (CNST) requires documentation of information listed as below as minimum:

- Who can perform the procedure?
- Assessment prior to performing the procedure
- Documentation of why the procedure is indicated
- Documentation of informed consent
- Ensuring effective analgesia
- Care of the bladder
- When to use sequential instruments
- When the procedure should be abandoned
- Care following OVB.

Proformas can improve record keeping after obstetric interventions[26] and would usefully be employed after OVB. An example of a proforma for OVB documentation is included within the RCOG Green-top Guideline for Operative Vaginal Delivery[7] and is reproduced above (Figure 8.2).

Conclusion

OVB can improve outcomes for mothers and their babies. However, its safe use requires accurate clinical assessment, skilled use of instruments, anticipation of potential complications and good communication. Training can improve all of these elements, to reduce preventable harm and, consequently, litigation.

References

1. Joint WHO/UNFPA/UNICEF World Bank Statement. *Reduction of Maternal Mortality*, Geneva: WHO, 1999;1.

2. Oliphant SS, Jones KA, Wang L, Bunker CH, Lowder JL. Trends over time with commonly performed obstetric and gynecologic inpatient procedures. *Obstet Gynecol* 2010;116:926–31.

3. Lumbiganon P, Laopaiboon M, Gülmezoglu AM, Souza JP, Taneepanichskul S, Ruyan P, et al. Method of delivery and pregnancy outcomes in Asia: the WHO global survey on maternal and perinatal health 2007–08. *Lancet* 2010;375:490–9.

4. Murphy DJ, Liebling RE, Verity L, Swingler R, Patel R. Early maternal and neonatal morbidity associated with operative delivery in second stage of labour: a cohort study. *Lancet* 2001;358:1203–7.

5. Walsh CA, Robson M, McAuliffe FM. Mode of delivery at term and adverse neonatal outcomes. *Obstet Gynecol* 2013;121:122–8.

6. Murphy DJ, Koh DK. Cohort study of the decision to delivery interval and neonatal outcome for emergency operative vaginal delivery. *Am J Obstet Gynecol* 2007;196:145 e1–7.

7. Royal College of Obstetricians and Gynaecologists. *Operative vaginal delivery*. Green-top Guideline No. 26. London: RCOG; 2011.

8. National Institute for Health and Care Excellence. *Intrapartum care: Care of healthy women and their babies during childbirth*. London: NICE; 2007.

9. Bahl R, Strachan B, Murphy DJ. Outcome of subsequent pregnancy three years after previous operative delivery in the second stage of labour: cohort study. *BMJ* 2004;328:311.

10. Jolly J, Walker J, Bhabra K. Subsequent obstetric performance related to primary mode of delivery. *BJOG* 1999;106:227–32.

11. Clark EA, Silver RM. Long-term maternal morbidity associated with repeat cesarean delivery. *Am J Obstet Gynecol* 2011;205 Suppl 6:S2–10.

12. O'Mahony F, Hofmeyr GJ, Menon V. Choice of instruments for assisted vaginal delivery. *Cochrane Database Syst Rev* 2010;(11):CD005455.

13. Johanson RB, Menon V. Vacuum extraction versus forceps for assisted vaginal delivery, *Cochrane Database Syst Rev*, 2004;(2):CD000224.

14. Burke N, Field K, Mujahid F, Morrison JJ, Use and safety of Kielland's forceps in current obstetric practice. *Obstet Gynecol* 2012;120:766–70.

15. NHS Litigation Authority. *Ten Years of Maternity Claims: An Analysis of NHS Litigation Authority Data*. London: NHSLA; 2012.

16. Patel RR, Murphy DJ. Forceps delivery in modern obstetric practice. *BMJ* 2004;328:1302–5.

17. Attilakos G, Sibanda T, Winter C, Johnson N, Draycott T. A randomised controlled trial of a new handheld vacuum extraction device. *BJOG* 2005;112:1510–5.

18. Royal College of Obstetricians and Gynaecologists. *The management of third- and fourth-degree perineal tears*. Green-top Guideline No. 29. London: RCOG; 2001.

19. McCandlish R, Bowler U, van Asten H, Berridge G, Winter C, Sames L, et al. A randomised controlled trial of care of the perineum during second stage of normal labour. *BJOG* 1998;105:1262–72.

20. Murphy DJ, Macleod M, Bahl R, Goyder K, Howarth L, Strachan B. A randomised controlled trial of routine versus restrictive use of episiotomy at operative vaginal delivery: a multicentre pilot study. *BJOG* 2008;115:1695–702; discussion 1702–3.

21. Andrews V, Sultan AH, Thakar R, Jones PW. Occult anal sphincter injuries – myth or reality? *BJOG* 2006;113:195–200.

22. Groom KM, Paterson-Brown S. Can we improve on the diagnosis of third degree tears? *Eur J Obstet Gynecol Reprod Biol* 2002;101:19–21.

23. Kirke P. Mothers' views of care in labour. *BJOG* 1980;87:1034–8.

24. Siassakos D, Bristowe K, Hambly H, Angouri J, Crofts JF, Winter C, et al. Team communication with patient actors: findings from a multisite simulation study. *Simul Healthc* 2011;6:143–9.

25. Crofts JF, Bartlett C, Ellis D, Winter C, Donald F, Hunt LP, Draycott TJ. Patient-actor perception of care: a comparison of obstetric emergency training using manikins and patient-actors. *Qual Saf Health Care* 2008;17:20–4.

26. Crofts JF, Bartlett C, Ellis D, Fox R, Draycott TJ. Documentation of simulated shoulder dystocia: accurate and complete? *BJOG*. 2008;115:1303–8.

Chapter 9
Analgesia and anaesthesia for operative vaginal birth

Rowena Pykett, George Bugg and David Levy

Key learning points

■ There are a number of techniques available to provide anaesthesia and analgesia for operative vaginal birth (OVB), each with benefits and drawbacks dependent on the situation.

■ An understanding of these techniques, in parallel with clinical assessment of the woman and scenario, will allow individualisation in each case.

This chapter deals with methods of analgesia and anaesthesia for OVB. Previous chapters have discussed the decision-making processes underpinning which type of birth is required and where to perform it; this chapter details the various types of analgesia and anaesthesia used in different situations.

OVB can be undertaken either in the labour room or in theatre. Estimation of the likelihood of vaginal birth proving successful is pivotal to informing decision making in terms of analgesic and anaesthetic requirements.

Assessment of the woman by an experienced obstetrician will determine whether a birth can be conducted safely in the labour room. If there is a material risk or failed operative vaginal birth requiring conversion to caesarean section, transfer to the operating theatre will be indicated.

The following points interact to influence the timing, location and instrument choice:

- efficacy of maternal effort and degree of descent with pushing
- station and position of the fetal head
- suspected fetal condition based on cardiotocography (CTG) monitoring and/or fetal blood sampling (FBS)
- analgesic requirements of the mother
- experience and confidence of the person conducting the birth.

Local anaesthetic infiltration

The use of local anaesthesia for low cavity and outlet OVB, where it is expected to be straightforward, can allow the procedure to be carried out in the labour suite.

The operator must be confident that the birth can be achieved without recourse to caesarean section. Based on the woman's rapport with both midwife and obstetrician and her tolerance of vaginal examinations, an estimation can be made of her likely analgesic requirement and whether she is likely to tolerate an operative vaginal birth under local anaesthesia alone.

Local anaesthesia has the advantages of wide availability and low cost. It is administered by the obstetrician attending the woman: an anaesthetist does not need to be available at the time. A local anaesthetic block will only relieve vaginal and perineal pain – there is no effect on the pain of uterine contractions.

Local anaesthetic pharmacology

Local anaesthetics are reversible membrane-stabilising drugs; they block the sodium channels in the nerve membrane, preventing depolarisation and transmission of nerve impulses. A number of local anaesthetic agents are available: lidocaine is the most widely used in obstetrics in the UK. Various local anaesthetic preparations have been investigated. A recent Cochrane review has concluded that there is little difference between them.[1]

Lidocaine administered by infiltration has an onset of 5–10 minutes and duration of around 45 minutes.[2] There is no demonstrable benefit in adding adrenaline to local anaesthesia for pudendal infiltration: adrenaline-containing solutions are not routinely used in the UK.[3] Bupivacaine should not be used on account of its potential for systemic toxicity.

Table 9.1 Symptoms and signs of local anaesthetic toxicity

Symptoms	Signs
Numbness of tongue or lips	Slurring of speech
Tinnitus	Drowsiness
Light-headedness	Convulsions
Anxiety	Cardiorespiratory arrest

Lidocaine 1% contains 10 mg lidocaine per 1 ml solution. The recommended maximum dose for infiltration is 3 mg/kg. For a 70 kg woman, a total of 210 mg is allowed, equivalent to a volume of 21 ml 1% lidocaine.

Local anaesthetic toxicity

Systemic toxicity can develop secondary to either direct accidental administration into an artery or vein, or systemic absorption via vascular tissues of an excessive administered dose. Toxicity affects primarily the central nervous and cardiovascular systems (Table 9.1).

It is important to maintain verbal communication with the woman to discern symptoms while injecting LA. Treatment of toxicity follows the general ABC principles of resuscitation with concurrent relief of aortocaval compression from the gravid uterus. Specific treatment for local anaesthesia-induced seizures or impending cardiac arrest is with Intralipid™ 20%. All labour wards should have an emergency box or trolley containing a LipidRescue™ box with instructions and equipment for infusion while resuscitation continues.[4]

Pudendal block and perineal infiltration

The majority of the innervation of the lower vagina, vulva and perineum is derived from the pudendal nerve (S2–4). The course of the nerve through the pelvis affords access for injection of local anaesthetic proximal to its division into terminal branches. The aim of blocking the pudendal nerve is to reduce sensation from the vagina and perineum sufficiently to allow low cavity and outlet OVB, including episiotomy and perineal repair.

Although pudendal block has been used for many decades, there is little evidence of its anaesthetic effectiveness. Literature searches have failed to identify any research over the last 50 years demonstrating the efficacy of pudendal block for OVB.[5] Allowing adequate time for the

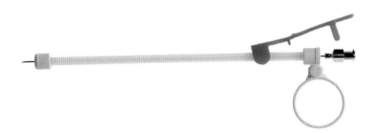

Figure 9.1 Rocket™ pudendal needle

local anaesthetic to work should provide better pain relief, providing fetal condition permits.

There are two techniques, outlined below, for paravaginal pudendal block that are recommended and used commonly in the UK. There are variations in continental Europe where the pudendal nerve is reached through the perineal skin.

- Draw up 20 ml 1% lidocaine without adrenaline into a syringe.
- Attach a special guarded pudendal needle (Figure 9.1) the aim of which is to limit the depth of penetration of the needle and reduce the risk of needlestick injuries.
- Between contractions, palpate the left ischial spine with the left hand, hold the syringe with the right hand and guide the guarded needle between the index and middle finger of the left hand (irrespective of operator handedness).
- **Technique 1** – rest the index finger on the ischial spine and run the guarded needle between the fingers until it rests on the tissues 1 cm medial and posterior to the ischial spine (Figure 9.2).
- **Technique 2** – rest the middle finger on the ischial spine with the index finger above it, run the guarded needle between the fingers until it rests on the tissues 1 cm medial and anterior to the ischial spine (Figure 9.3).
- Unhook the needle guard and insert the needle 1 cm into the tissues adjacent to the anticipated course of the pudendal nerve.
- Large pudendal vessels run close to the nerve. It is very important to aspirate once the needle is in place. If blood is aspirated, re-site the needle.
- Inject 7 ml of anaesthetic, then guard the needle and withdraw.
- Repeat the procedure on the opposite side, changing the hand used to palpate the ischial spine and hold the syringe.
- Finally, inject the remaining 6 ml of local anaesthetic into the perineum in a radial pattern from the posterior fourchette, again remembering to aspirate before injection to avoid injecting anaesthetic directly into the bloodstream.

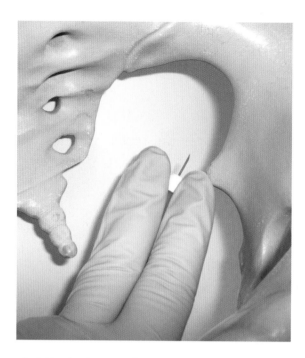

Figure 9.2 Technique 1 for paravaginal pudendal block

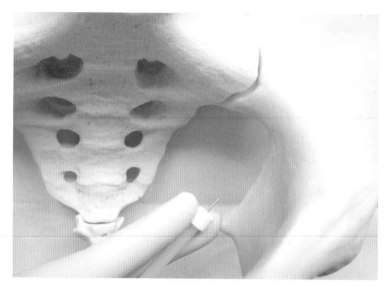

Figure 9.3 Technique 2 for paravaginal pudendal block

Occasionally the fetal head may be so low in the pelvis that palpating the ischial spines is impossible. In this scenario it would be unusual to require OVB. Perineal infiltration alone with 1% lidocaine 20 ml will permit adequate episiotomy. This method of perineal infiltration would also be appropriate for a birth requiring episiotomy alone.

While not universally performed, it is advisable to test the effectiveness of the block. This can be achieved by pinching the skin of the posterior fourchette with the operator's index finger and thumb. However, as the need for OVB is usually urgent, there is rarely time to rectify inadequate anaesthesia.

Complications

Carried out as described, a pudendal block is generally a safe procedure with few complications. The risk of needlestick injury in the course of this blind procedure should be minimised by gaining familiarity with the instrument. The potential exists for laceration from inadequate guarding of the needle and the formation of haematoma if the pudendal vessels are punctured. There are case reports of infection and abscess formation caused by inoculation of bacteria from the vagina. These conditions usually respond to conservative treatment. There is also potential for pudendal neuralgia if the nerve is traumatised, but no obstetric cases have been reported.

If there is any suspicion of accidental fetal injection a neonatologist should be forewarned. Neonatal signs include hypotonia, seizures and cardiorespiratory compromise.[6]

Regional blockade

Neuraxial regional blockade is effected by injection of local anaesthetic and/or opioid into the epidural and/or subarachnoid spaces, blocking sensory nerves as they enter the spinal cord.

Epidural and spinal anaesthesia are used on the labour ward for a number of reasons. Epidural analgesia is often used for pain relief during labour, with the advantage of providing anaesthesia for OVB in the room. Additionally, epidural top-up can be used for trial of OVB in theatre with possibility of recourse to caesarean section if unsuccessful.

The sensory innervation of the uterus and cervix extends from T10 to L1; innervation of the vagina, vulva and perineum is derived from S2 to S4 nerve roots. Regional analgesia for labour or OVB requires abolition of sensation from these levels in order to provide adequate pain relief. However, dermatomal anaesthetic level to T4–5 is needed for adequate anaesthesia for CS – to block sensation from the abdominal peritoneum and viscera.

Single-shot spinal anaesthesia is generally not used for pain relief in labour due to its limited duration, but has a vital role in providing anaesthesia for a trial of OVB in theatre.

Table 9.2 Features and comparison of epidural and spinal anaesthetic

Feature	Epidural	Spinal
Onset of block	Up to 30 minutes	Within 5 minutes
Duration of action	Can be extended	~90 minutes
Efficacy of block	Possibly incomplete	Usually complete
Drug requirement	Large, risks systemic local anaesthetic toxicity	Small (one-seventh of epidural dose)
Technique	Infusion or repeated top-up	Usually one shot
Headache	None unless accidental dural puncture	Rare, related to needle size and design
Hypotension	Uncommon	Universal – requires fluid/vasopressor

When implementing a regional anaesthetic technique for OVB, there is a compromise to be made between impairment of the woman's ability to push (reduced muscle power) versus adequacy of CS anaesthesia if conversion is required. A forceps birth does not necessarily require any maternal effort, but the use of vacuum to assist birth usually requires co-ordination with maternal effort. There is a place for a less dense top-up of epidural anaesthesia for a vacuum birth with a caveat that further time is required to provide anaesthesia for caesarean section if vaginal birth proves unsuccessful.

Combined doses of local anaesthetic and opioid reduce the total quantity of each drug required to provide adequate analgesia.[7] Table 9.2 compares epidural and spinal anaesthesia.

Provision of regional analgesia and anaesthesia requires the immediate availability of an experienced anaesthetist and should be available in UK consultant-led units. Contraindications to regional analgesia are outlined in Table 9.3 and Table 9.4 outlines the complications.

Table 9.3 Contraindications to regional analgesia, with associated reasons

Contraindication	Reason
Refusal by woman	Legal claim
Lack of sufficient staff for continuous care	Delayed recognition of maternal or fetal compromise
Uncorrected anticoagulation or coagulopathy	Vertebral canal haematoma
Local or systemic sepsis	Vertebral canal abscess
Hypovolaemia or active haemorrhage	Cardiovascular collapse attributable to sympathetic blockade

Table 9.4 Complications of regional anaesthesia

Risk	Event	Treatment
Accidental dural puncture	Accidental puncture of the meninges when siting epidural Leakage of cerebrospinal fluid can cause severe postural headache	Epidural blood patch (epidural injection of woman's own blood) best undertaken at 24–48 hours Follow up until symptom free
Total spinal	Large dose of local anaesthetic, intended for the epidural space, reaches the subarachnoid space Block reaching cervical segments will impair diaphragmatic innervation	Emergency tracheal intubation and treatment of hypotension Caesarean birth of the baby, urgency dependent on fetal monitoring
Local anaesthetic toxicity	See 'local anaesthetic infiltration'	

Epidural analgesia

Epidural analgesia is commonly provided in response to maternal request during the active first stage of labour. Alternatively, it may be jointly recommended by the anaesthetist and obstetrician anticipating a technically difficult anaesthetic in a woman at high risk of requiring OVB or caesarean section, for example an obese woman who has developed gestational diabetes with a high estimated fetal weight. It is rarely used de novo for OVB unless an underlying maternal condition (e.g. severe aortic stenosis) contraindicates the more rapid onset of spinal anaesthesia. Such women should be reviewed in an antenatal obstetric anaesthetic clinic where these challenges can be considered and appropriate plans formulated.

Labour epidural analgesia is associated with an increased risk of OVB although the chance of caesarean section is not influenced.[8]

The following steps are undertaken:

- Discussion with woman and informed consent
- Fetal and maternal monitoring
- Recent full blood count checked if necessary, intravenous access, fluids infusing at slow rate (e.g. 500 ml Hartmann's solution over 6 hours)
- Aseptic technique – hat, mask, gown, hand washing, gloves, antiseptic preparation of woman's back, sterile drapes
- Epidural needle (Tuohy needle) and loss-of-resistance syringe assembled
- Interspinous spaces palpated
- Local anaesthetic injected into skin
- Epidural needle advanced through the skin, subcutaneous tissues and ligamentum flavum
- Aspirate syringe to exclude placement in blood vessel or subarachnoid space
- Epidural catheter threaded via needle into epidural space
- Catheter secured in place
- Loading dose of opioid and/or local anaesthetic, followed by continuous or patient-controlled infusion of the same drug mixture.

A bilateral block of cold sensation to T10 (just above the umbilicus) should relieve the pain of uterine contractions. Block above T6 should prompt the epidural infusion to be stopped until the block regresses to T10.

When use of an existing labour epidural is planned for trial of OVB, the block must be sufficient to allow recourse to immediate caesarean section if vaginal birth proves unsuccessful. Once a decision is made for trial of OVB, the anaesthetist should be informed immediately in order that epidural top-up can be expedited. Conversion of labour epidural analgesia to surgical anaesthesia takes 15–20 minutes. Beginning the top-up in the labour room before transfer to theatre has the advantage of reducing the time to achieve surgical anaesthesia, but incurs the risks associated with minimal physiological monitoring during transfer to the operating theatre, e.g. hypotension and fetal compromise.

Single-shot spinal anaesthesia

In contrast to a large-gauge epidural needle (which facilitates passage of an epidural catheter) a finer gauge, tapered spinal needle is used for meningeal puncture and direct injection into the cerebrospinal fluid (CSF). If hyperbaric (denser than CSF) bupivacaine is used, the dose might be varied according to gestation. The addition of opioids can reduce the incidence of visceral pain.

Spinal anaesthesia is used for a trial of OVB in theatre where there is no or inadequate pre-existing epidural analgesia and there is a chance of recourse to caesarean section.

The block afforded by single-shot spinal anaesthesia develops faster than an epidural top-up. Surgical anaesthesia is achieved in 5–10 minutes. However, it can cause a sudden fall in blood pressure, with the potential for diminution of uteroplacental perfusion. Care must always be taken to minimise aortocaval compression by left-lateral tilt. The obstetrician must be mindful of the potential requirement for quick birth if there is evidence of fetal compromise, and should not leave theatre after institution of spinal anaesthesia.

The obstetrician must bear in mind that surgical anaesthesia is generally limited to 90 minutes, and that there is no facility to prolong the anaesthetic block. Caesarean section following unsuccessful OVB carries an increased risk of complications, especially postpartum haemorrhage. There should be good communication throughout between surgeon and anaesthetist so that adequate adjuvant analgesia can be given to keep the woman comfortable, and an awareness that general anaesthesia may be required if there is uncontrolled blood loss and the surgery becomes protracted.

Combined spinal–epidural techniques

Less commonly used, combined spinal–epidural (CSE) analgesia and anaesthesia have the advantages of a rapid onset of spinal block with the flexibility afforded by an epidural catheter. An initial dose of subarachnoid local anaesthetic and opioid can be supplemented by further doses of drugs via the epidural catheter.

Such a technique could be useful if a surgical birth was anticipated to be complicated, for instance an elective caesarean section after multiple previous abdominal surgeries.

General anaesthesia

General anaesthesia may be required if an unsuccessful OVB necessitates caesarean section and the regional block is inadequate. A much less common scenario would be where an OVB under local anaesthesia was thought to be possible but has been unsuccessful, and regional anaesthesia was absolutely contraindicated for any reason.

This is usually a tense situation for all involved, and good communication is vital. The safety of the mother is of utmost importance; time and patience is vital for a safe general anaesthetic even when there are significant fetal concerns.

The main maternal risks of general anaesthesia are airway problems such as failed intubation, aspiration of gastric contents and anaphylaxis to the neuromuscular blocking drug succinylcholine. General anaesthetic drugs are innocuous to the fetus in the long term although transient respiratory depression, requirement for active resuscitation and low Apgar scores are more common after general anaesthesia compared with regional blockade, regardless of events prior to caesarean section.

Concerns following birth

When a birth has been performed under regional anaesthesia, it is easy to neglect subsequent postpartum analgesia as the woman will be comfortable at the time of birth. It is common to give diclofenac per rectum following OVB (provided there are no contraindications), and to prescribe regular analgesia as appropriate for the following days.

Venous thromboembolism (VTE) has been highlighted as a leading cause of maternal mortality in successive triennial mortality reports and must be considered following OVB. Proformas for scoring women's individual risk factors are recommended. The increased risk of VTE following midcavity OVB versus low cavity birth is reflected by an increased score.[9]

References

1. Novikova N, Cluver C. Local anaesthetic nerve block for pain management in labour. *Cochrane Database Syst Rev* 2012;(4):CD009200.

2. Palmer CM, D'Angelo R, Paech MJ. *Obstetric Anaesthesia*. Oxford: Oxford University Press; 2011.

3. Schierup L, Schmidt JF, Torp Jensen A, Rye BA. Pudendal block in vaginal deliveries. Mepivacaine with and without epinephrine. *Acta Obstet Gynecol Scand* 1988;67:195–7.

4. LipidRescue. Available at: http://lipidrescue.org/ (accessed 22 June 2012).

5. Scudamore JH, Yates MJ. Pudendal block—a misnomer? *Lancet* 1966;1:23–4.

6. Sinclair JC, Fox HA, Lentz JF, Fuld GL, Murphy J. Intoxication of the fetus by a local anesthetic. *N Engl J Med* 1965;273:1173.

7. Chestnut D, Polley S, Lawrence CT, Wong CA. *Chestnut's Obstetric Anaesthesia – Principles and Practice 4th edition*. Mosby; 2009.

8. Royal College of Obstetricians and Gynaecologists. *Operative vaginal delivery*. Green-top Guideline No. 26. London: RCOG; 2011.

9. Royal College of Obstetricians and Gynaecologists. *Reducing the risk of thrombosis and embolism in pregnancy and the puerperium*. Green-top Guideline No. 37a. London: RCOG; 2009.

Index

Note: page numbers in *italics* refer to figures, tables and flow charts